TEACHING
IN AND BEYOND
PANDEMIC TIMES

Editors:
Jonathan D Jansen & Theola Farmer-Phillips

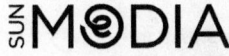

Teaching In and Beyond Pandemic Times

Published by African Sun Media under the SUN MeDIA imprint
Place of publication: Stellenbosch, South Africa

All rights reserved

Copyright © 2021 African Sun Media and the editors

The editors and the publisher have made every effort to obtain permission for and acknowledge the use of copyrighted material. Refer all enquiries to the publisher.

No part of this book may be reproduced or transmitted in any form or by any electronic, photographic or mechanical means, including photocopying and recording on record, tape or laser disk, on microfilm, via the Internet, by e-mail, or by any other information storage and retrieval system, without prior written permission by the publisher.

Views reflected in this publication are not necessarily those of the publisher.

First edition 2021

ISBN 978-1-928314-01-1
ISBN 978-1-928314-49-3 (e-book)
https://doi.org/10.52779/9781928314493

Set in Myriad Pro Light 10/14

Cover design, typesetting and production by African Sun Media
Cover photograph © Nirode Bramdaw

SUN MeDIA is an imprint of African Sun Media. Academic and general works are published under this imprint in print and electronic formats.

This publication can be ordered from:
orders@africansunmedia.co.za
Takealot: bit.ly/2monsfl
Google Books: bit.ly/2k1Uilm
africansunmedia.store.it.si *(e-books)*
Amazon Kindle: amzn.to/2ktL.pkL

Visit africansunmedia.co.za for more information.

Contents

Key acronyms used in this book vii

The 2020 academic timeline for public schools ix

Introduction and orientation to the book 1
Jonathan D Jansen & Theola Farmer-Phillips

1 A tribute to South Africa's teachers 7
  David J Millar

2 A dedicatory poem 11
  Erin Chothia-Lakay

3 Perspective as co-editor of this book, and
  as a practising teacher 15
  Theola Farmer-Phillips

4 Teacher stories about pandemic teaching 19
  4.1 Pressure 19
  4.2 Pedagogy 26
  4.3 (P)reparation 38
  4.4 Pioneers 47
  4.5 Poverty 68
  4.6 Privilege 85
  4.7 Perspective (novice teachers, older teachers) 99
  4.8 Parents, Parent teachers 111
  4.9 Peer teaching 126
  4.10 Perseverance 136
  4.11 Pastoral care 141

5 What do we learn from the teacher stories in this book?
  Ten lessons for a post-pandemic school system 149
  Jonathan D Jansen & Theola Farmer-Phillips

Resources on pandemic school teaching for further
reading and research 159

Contributing authors 161

Key acronyms used in this book

Acronym	Stands for	Meaning
ATPs	Annual Teaching Plans	The document outlines the specific teaching topics, teaching timeframe and assessment requirements per subject/grade.
CA	Curriculum Advisor/Subject Advisor	Specialist in the education field who plays a vital advisory and supportive role for teachers.
CAPS	Curriculum Assessment Policy Statements	The curriculum policy governing the education of learners in Grades R to 12.
CTLI	The Cape Teaching and Leadership Institution	An institution that offers professional development courses on an in-service basis to educators in the Western Cape.
DBE	Department of Basic Education	The national department of education concerned with schools.
ECD	Early Childhood Development	The years preceding formal schooling in Grade 1.
EGRA	Early Grade Reading Development	A diagnostic reading test, done in the foundation phase (Grades 1 to 3).
GET	General Education and Training	The education and training provided from Grades R to 9 at school level and includes Adult Basic Education and Training.
ICT	Information and Communication Technologies	Generally used in this book to refer to all the technology platforms for teaching and learning.
LMS	Learning Management Systems	Often used in reference to e-learning platforms.
Nodal schools	Schools chosen to teach a specialist subject and to be a resource school for other schools in the area	Such as Marine Sciences, which is not widely offered in the standard curriculum.
NSC	National Senior Certificate	The certificate issued at the end of Grade 12 final examinations, sometimes referred to as "matric".

Acronym	Stands for	Meaning
OBE	Outcomes-Based Education	The outcomes-driven approach to education adopted by the new South African government in 1998.
PoAs	Programme of Assessment	A scheduled guide with specific details pertaining to school-based assessment for learners.
PPE	Personal Protective Equipment	Equipment meant to protect from infection, such as gloves, masks, etc.
PSP	Primary Science Programme	A non-profit organisation that offers training and mentorship to educators, especially newly qualified educators.
SBA	School-Based Assessment	A range of assessments being undertaken at school level, leading up to an examination.
SMT	School Management Team	The principal, deputy principals and departmental heads of a school.
SOP	Standard Operating Procedure	A document by Department of Basic Education that outlines standard procedures and protocols to be followed in the prevention, containment, and management of Covid-19 in schools.
TREP	Temporary Revised Education Plans	A detailed plan which outlines the standard operating procedure in the prevention and management of Covid-19 infections at school level.
WCED	Western Cape Education Department	The government department in the Western Cape, South Africa, responsible for primary and secondary education.
YIP	Years in Phase	A learner who was retained in a specific phase, yet is still displaying difficulty in performing at the expected level. A learner may only be retained once in every four years.

The 2020 academic timeline for public schools

Term 1: 15 January–18 March 2020	
15 January 2020	All learners at school as per normal pre-Covid
18 March 2020	Schools closed by presidential announcement
20 March 2020	Initial end-of-term date
Term 2: 1 June–24 July 2020	
1 June 2020	Grades 7 and 12 all return to school
6 July 2020	ECD, Grades R, 1, 2, 3 and 6 return to school
24 July 2020	School closes
Term 3: 3 August–23 October 2020	
3 August 2020	Grade 12 learners return to school
11 August 2020	Grade 7 learners return to school
24 August 2020	Grades R, 1, 2, 3, 4 and 6 return to Primary School Grades 9, 10 and 11 return to High School
31 August 2020	Grades 5 and 8 return to school
23 October 2020	School closes
Term 4: 2 November–15 December 2020	
Grades R to 12 return to school	

Introduction and orientation to the book

Since the 2020 publication of *Learning under Lockdown*, a focus on children's experience of pandemic learning, there has been a stream of requests from South African teachers for a complementary edition, perhaps called *Teaching under Lockdown*. While these two educational processes are inextricably linked, teaching is not learning, and learning is not teaching. Teaching may or may not result in learning and we know that learning can happen with or without teaching. We, therefore, wanted to do a "deep dive" into teaching during the pandemic, and especially during that period (the hard lockdown) when teachers and learners were physically separated from each other.

The experience of learners captured in *Learning under Lockdown* was at once despairing and hopeful. We read stories of distress but also resilience. In that collection, we saw the inequalities of school education laid bare; we could no longer look away as a minority of children experienced a seamless transition from face-to-face teaching to online learning while the majority were immediately cut off from those three vital instructional resources: teachers, texts, and time. Written in the first person, the more than 400 children's stories detailed the emotions of caring and coping; the hard choices that had to be made between data or bread; and the tough negotiations within the family about the use of living spaces as learning and working spaces under lockdown.

But what about the teachers? At the time of composing this book, there were very few systematic accounts of the experiences of teaching during the lockdown. Most of what was available in writing came in the form of teacher blogs and other online commentaries, stories in professional journals, and newspaper articles on teacher experiences working from home. In the heat of pandemic teaching, few writings at the time linked current experiences to future trends. We wanted to do more by both presenting 65 stories in a structured way and then analysing the experiences of those teachers from what they tell us about the present (e.g., the deep inequalities and how they frame teaching under pandemic conditions) and the future (e.g., the inevitability of hybrid teaching).

As editors, though we had some of our starting questions, we were always conscious of the need to let the stories speak for themselves, that is, to allow other questions to emerge from the teacher accounts as submitted. Our initial questions included the ones below.

How did teachers maintain, or at least try to maintain, contact with their charges at a distance? What were the inventive ways in which teachers reached out to children who had no reliable access to data and devices? How did younger and often more tech-savvy teachers make the transition to online learning compared to older teachers for whom the technology could be expected to be a serious challenge? What do we know about the emotional lives of teachers, especially when they had to return to school as the lockdown eased? Under these conditions, how did schools deploy their teachers when their colleagues with comorbidities were allowed to remain at home?

We knew, however, that a book on pandemic teaching would hold limited value if we only told the story about teachers and teaching at the height of the Covid-19 crisis. Of course, capturing that period in time is no doubt important for the historical record and to provide generations of readers and researchers with a rich source of data for the moment. But we also wanted to examine the lessons learnt from pandemic teaching for what it means to teach (and learn) once this crisis is behind us. What did we learn about the consequences of inequality for this particular mode of teaching? Which compensatory resources are more effective in delivering teaching under the particular resource constraints imposed by a pandemic? What new forms of partnership, amongst teachers themselves and between teachers and department officials such as curriculum advisors, can be built on in the future? And what kinds of teaching infrastructures need to be put in place for possible future lockdowns, as epidemiologists predict?

To gain answers to these and related questions, we used methods that proved valuable in the study of learning under lockdown. We used our extensive social media networks, principally Facebook and Twitter, to invite teachers from the nine provinces to submit their stories about teaching under lockdown. A set of guiding questions were distributed so that all the submissions spoke to more or less the same set of interests.

For example, we want to know how the pandemic lockdown impacted their pedagogies or modes of teaching; what was different and what was the same from pre-pandemic times? We wanted to know about the effects of lockdown on their emotional, psychological, and mental lives and how that, in turn, impacted their teaching. We asked about creative or inventive ways of teaching remotely. What about the relationships with and expectations from parents as co-teachers, in some respects, of children separated from school for more than three months? And we were curious about the roles of curriculum advisors and other departmental officials in relation to subject teaching?

At the same time, it was important to us not to impose too tight a structure on the teacher stories, for then we would lose the many creative ways of writing in which our authors could give expression to teaching under lockdown. As a result, we received poems as well as traditional narrative writing, shorter and longer stories, straightforward, factual accounts and funny ones. The stories of music teachers carried a very different tonal quality to those of the Science teachers; the concerns about teaching new foundation phase learners were expressed differently amongst those teachers preparing young people for the all-important 'matric' examination.

Yet all of these stories of pandemic teaching give the public unique insight into what was often invisible to the outside world – the enormous burden that teachers carried through the extended lockdown.

Once the stories were received, mainly via email attachment, we selected the ones for publication based on the following criteria: relevance to the invited theme (pandemic teaching); focus and coherence; innovative insight or unusual understanding; quality of writing; exceptional commitment; and diversity of contexts. Stories containing mundane detail about teaching and that were repetitive in relation to other qualifying stories were not included. We also excluded stories that were little more than bitter attacks on the provincial department(s) of education rather than an illumination of teaching under historical conditions of constraint.

Then the stories were classified or categorised under specific themes that emerged from our analysis of each submission. Those themes are pressure, pedagogy, preparation, pioneers, poverty, privilege, and perspective. Each theme draws attention to a salient concern in the telling of a cluster of stories that together convey a sense of what it means to teach in the middle of a life-threatening crisis.

We edited most of the stories in part for coherence with the other stories and in part because of structure and grammar. Our guiding principle as editors was one of non-interference except in the case of obvious editorial corrections or style that was completely out of synch with the other stories. Even so, some teachers objected. They wanted the story told in their language, whatever the perceived shortcomings from the perspective of the editors. In all cases where objections were raised, we relented in favour of the teachers and kept their stories as submitted.

It is important to stress at this point that ours is *not* a standard academic book with dutiful references to theory, literature reviews and methodology. A scholarly account of teaching based on teacher stories can take many forms. We choose the narrative form because teacher stories are deeply personal, fluid, authentic, vivid, evocative, intense, honest, intimate and revealing of the very human actions at the heart of pandemic teaching. They are not constrained by a priori theories or pressed into particular regimens of method. The teacher stories speak for themselves. From these stories, we draw the policy implications for post-pandemic teaching.

One problem encountered in the open solicitation of teacher stories was the question of anonymity. Some teachers did not want to have their names (or even the names of their schools) made known in the stories. We respected requests for anonymity and marked those stories with an asterisk. It is not clear to us what the reasons were that some teachers requested secrecy given the purpose of the book – to shine a revealing light on teachers and teaching in a pandemic in ways that offer insights for post-pandemic schools and classrooms. What is clear is that we do not have a culture in our public schools where all professional teachers feel that they can talk openly about their lived experiences without repercussions.

Our purpose was always to foreground teachers' accounts of their lives. For example, in the process of telling, these stories emphatically refute a common misperception on the outside – that teachers were on an extended holiday enjoying rest and recreation while the children were couped up at home. Nothing could be further from the truth. As you read these stories, you will encounter heartbreak and longing, frustration and fear, care, and commitment, all rolled into one.

In other words, the collection of stories will reveal that pandemic teaching unfolded within a context that made them vulnerable and valued at the same time. Vulnerable, in that they were frontline workers receiving children in managed numbers, at a time when so little was known about the virus and its transmission within confined spaces such as classrooms. Colleagues fell ill and some died. The effects of such loss on teachers were often terrifying. Valued, because every parent knew that the difference between progression and failure in a year of unprecedented disruption was what that teacher was able to accomplish between home and school.

As we reflected on the stories, we learnt so much about the act of teaching itself, especially under crisis conditions. We saw extraordinary flexibility on the part of teachers as the rules changed for both health assurance and curriculum scope. The uncertainty caused significant frustration amongst teachers, but they made the necessary adjustments and readjustments as required. These were unprecedented times; planning was never an exact science.

In these contexts, South African teachers emerge as heroes and this book of stories is intended to honour them, especially those educators who succumbed to Covid-19. Our nation owes them a great, great debt of gratitude.

What's next? We now have teachers' stories alongside learners' stories, but there is a missing element that completes the loop of teaching and learning in pandemic times. Expect the third book in the trilogy to carry the title 'Parenting during lockdown', or more precisely, 'Parent-teaching during the lockdown'. Parents have always been involved to a greater or lesser extent in the education of their children. But the pandemic made that role both explicit and vital for learning from home over long periods of time.

Some schools literally taught segments of a lesson plan to parents online in order for them to teach the same content to their children, using methods the teacher would have used in the classroom. This book will also examine parent-teaching across social classes on the presumption that the social and cultural capital of middle-class parents gives them more resources to draw on in supporting the learning of their children from home; for working-class parents, those resources are not as readily available even if the commitment to their children's learning is the same. In short, what actually happened with respect to parent-teaching in the lockdown period for different families, including those where the parent was a schoolteacher?

This middle book in the trilogy, however, focuses sharply on what we learnt about teachers and teaching during the pandemic and what those lessons offer us for post-pandemic times. We now invite you to enjoy these teacher stories in their own words.

JONATHAN D JANSEN
Stellenbosch University

THEOLA FARMER-PHILLIPS
Yellowwood Primary School

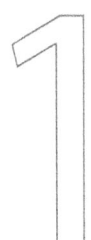

A tribute to South Africa's teachers

David J Millar

*Former District Superintendent / Director
Western Cape Education Department*

A quick search online will bring up pages upon pages of developers rhapsodising on the merits of their laptops and computer offerings. Inevitably, "core", "memory ram", "professional", "harness the power", "designed for groundbreaking performance", "all day battery life", and "2-year onsite warranty" appear above the "add to cart" choice bar.

Teaching during lockdown

Sounds to me like much of South Africa's teaching corps during lockdown, except that our teachers have a lifetime guarantee! In keeping with an IT-related metaphor, let's add the term 'commitment device' (pardon the pun) to the many descriptions of teachers during lockdown. They were grounded, flexible and purposeful. Their innovative agency made them resilient energisers as they built up collaborative networks in an unfamiliar space. Overnight. Literally.

Teachers discover early that their love of children draws them to teaching. For so many, their own love of learning makes them passionate about teaching. Many teachers I know were inspired by a teacher earlier in their own education who had a positive impact on them. Now they inspire.

When the pandemic hit, teachers had to dig deep as they took several dizzying breaths and then got on with the job. They had honed their skills for decades in front of a class and then, suddenly, had to develop a whole new set of skills on the spot. Trial and error. They expected that it would be tough, planned for it and did their best to make peace with it. They gave themselves time, and permission, to figure it out.

Of course, not all had the luxury to enter a virtual world – but there was nothing 'virtual' about the role. Defining 'virtual' is not difficult. It refers to something not physically existing as such but made by computer software to appear to do so. It was anything but! When it came to our teachers, they not only showed up; they stepped up physically. Much of the space may have been virtual, but it was real teachers who crowded the extra mile to take the hands of their learners.

Do not forget the teachers who stood in car parks at schools, in communities with no technology or access to the Internet, handing out 'drive-by-pick-up-and-go' curriculum packs, pre-prepared and packaged, while simultaneously handing out food parcels to indigent and vulnerable children. Parents would queue to take delivery of resources that kept their children busy. Perhaps this was the first time many parents actually got to see their child's teachers in the 'trenches' of education – albeit in a car park wearing a mask!

The dynamic and industrious way in which the teaching profession shared their newly found skills, knowledge and expertise is nothing short of miraculous. Teachers were energised and engaged, despite the anxiety that a global pandemic brought. Every single mindset vibe was, "I've got this." In a Ted Talk over a decade ago, the late Rita Pierson said, "We can do this … because we are educators! We are born to make a difference."

I can imagine that every teacher expected to deliver their lessons with perfection, but the reality was that they were just trying their best to get their classes taught – other people's children. Yet, most teachers had to take on various roles during lockdown isolation, including that of wife, husband, mother and father at the same time as being mentor, counsellor and 'Zoom controller'.

Teachers' lives were disrupted, much like Covid-19 disrupted life as we know it. Yet, they never flinched. Teachers did their best each day. Many had to switch from a chalkboard to a Zoom call overnight. Watching some of the online lessons that leaked onto the Internet showed teachers' exceptional communication, listening and organisational skills, and wicked sense of humour. It was refreshing to see and provided us with a glimpse into the real lives of teachers. Their strong work ethic, patience and friendly attitude made them our (s)heroes.

It was Charles Darwin who noted: "In the long history of humankind, those who learnt to collaborate and improvise most effectively have prevailed." While Covid-19 forced our entire population into lockdown, with a stuttering stop-start-stop-start to education, teachers scrambled to redesign their teaching and learning to allow learners of all ages to learn at home. It reimagined what learning looks like in the 21st century.

We cannot predict what technologies will be ascendant in future despite the 'OECD 2030 Future of Education and Skills Project' indicating the necessity of replacing old educational standards with an educational framework that combines knowledge with the 21st-century skills of creativity, critical thinking, communication and collaboration. In South Africa, this is still far off. What we can predict, though, is that teachers will prevail as the purveyors of hope to generations of South Africa's youth.

Conventional wisdom holds that motivation is the key to habit change. Any look at how teachers embraced change during Covid-19 lockdown challenges this wisdom. Teachers changed their entire teaching modalities out of necessity. Not motivation. They knew what their learners needed. If ever there was a time when teachers did it out of sheer love and concern for their charges, it was during lockdown. In addition, if the 'Law of Least Effort' states that people will naturally gravitate towards the option that requires the least amount of work when it comes to teachers teaching during the pandemic, one can dispel that as a myth.

If there is a silver lining to this all, it is that Covid-19 has resulted in public recognition of schools' essential caretaking role in society, and parents' gratitude for teachers, their skills, and their invaluable role in learners' well-being. Let us acknowledge the hard work, passion and extraordinary effort of our teachers during lockdown. It is right to show gratitude for our teachers' social and emotional support, compassion, encouragement and connection.

Teachers sell hope. They choose to teach, because they want to be vessels of hope and courage. Despite great adversity, they adjusted their sails, forged ahead and guided their learners in unchartered waters.

Schools closed, but teaching and learning did not.

#THANKYOUTEACHER.

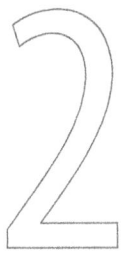

A dedicatory poem

Erin Chothia-Lakay

Fairbairn College
Goodwood

Behind closed doors

Behind closed doors, I read
I read articles about the stats of this terrifying pandemic
I scroll my newsfeed relentlessly
I read … another teacher has contracted this virus …
I read … another teacher has lost their life to this virus …
I read … scheduled media briefings …
I read … postponed media briefings …
I read … zoom meetings by the powers that be about MY future
I read … all the while remaining mute about how I really feel
Behind closed doors, I read

Behind closed doors, I am angry
I am angered by the fact that despite my best intentions I am part of the system that is failing us
I am angered that I am held ransom by my pay-check
I must bite my tongue, be strong, and do my job under the current pressures if I want to continue to provide for my family
I am angry that I feel like I must pay for "all the holidays and little work I do" with my well-being
I am angered by the lack of empathy and the disregard for the fact that I too am only human
I am angered by the fact that even if I wanted to, I cannot walk away
Behind closed doors, I am angry

Behind closed doors, I am fearful
I fear that speaking my truth could result in losing my livelihood
I fear the eruption of emotions I've been suppressing
I fear the threat this virus poses to all of us
I fear that mine will be the next family affected
I fear that my children will grow up without their mom because I am the high risk one in our household
I fear that I will be replaced in a heartbeat and the pain of their loss will linger long after the sent flowers have wilted
So, Behind closed doors, I am fearful

Behind closed doors, I'm no longer a clown
I no longer have to perfect the art of juggling …
No juggling working as if I have no family and parenting as if I have no work
I no longer have my heavily made-up face to disguise that I am battling to keep up with keeping everyone happy
My costume and clown suit replaced by the plain clothes of despair
Behind closed doors, I am no longer a clown

Behind closed doors, I am no longer a robot
I no longer have to put on my mechanical brave face for the learners because I am instructed to not let them see my fear or anxiety
I no longer have to hold my breath as I walk the passages with my plastered robot smile
I no longer have to go about my daily business as if I'm not falling apart inside
Behind closed doors, I am no longer a robot

Behind closed doors, I am restless
My mind races
Despite my exhaustion, my body won't switch off
I sacrifice sleep for planning, prepping, late-night WhatsApps from learners, creating online learning material, restless toddlers and worry
My stomach in knots as I reflect on the day that has passed and contemplate the day that lies ahead
My mind races
Behind closed doors, I am restless

Behind closed doors, I am guilt-ridden
Nine weeks at home left me itching to get back into the classroom … I was eager … knowing in my heart of hearts that it was too soon
I am guilt-ridden … torn between "let's get in there and get things going" and "I didn't sign up for this"
I am guilt-ridden for not acknowledging how I truly feel and not speaking out
Behind closed doors, I am guilt-ridden

Behind closed doors, I weep
Unable to hold back as it all bubbles to the surface
I weep for job losses, families without a roof over their heads or food on the table, those who are ill and those who have succumbed
I weep for the apprehensive faces in the classroom staring back at me every day
I weep for the ones I am unable to reach due to lack of resources
I weep because with each passing day it gets closer to home
I weep for my little 3 & 4-year-old who have to soldier to school every day because this Mommy can't home school
I weep because I have no choice, no say and no other option
Yes, Behind closed doors, I weep

Behind closed doors, I am discouraged
Unable to give any facet of my life the best of me as I'm pouring from an empty cup
Disheartened by the reality that following my passion has now turned into dismay
Saddened by the reality that I am just an employee number on a payroll … a lamb to the slaughter … a sitting duck
Behind closed doors, I am discouraged

Behind closed doors, I pray
I pray for courage … the courage I need to confront the fear that envelops me
I pray for strength … the strength I need to fight my exhausted body and keep going
I pray for peace … to calm the raging storm inside me
I pray for release … because holding onto all I feel will leave a bitter taste of this profession in my mouth
I give thanks … for I know that He is and always has been at the helm
Behind closed doors, I pray

Behind closed doors, I am human
Erin
Daughter
Sister
Wife
Mommy
Aunt
Friend
Teacher
Colleague
HUMAN
Behind closed doors, I am human

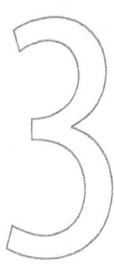

Perspective as co-editor of this book, and as a practising teacher

THEOLA FARMER-PHILLIPS

*Yellowwood Primary School
Western Cape*

> "Driving to school and going back home was like moving between different levels of lockdown."

Prayer kept me sane in this time. As positive cases and the death toll shot upwards, it finally hit me: we need to teach through this pandemic. I never thought I would live in, let alone teach and lead through, a pandemic. At school, we were constantly reminded that we are the school management team (SMT), the select few called upon to lead. The powerful phrase, "When a crisis reveals itself, leadership shows up", lingered with me. School leaders were about to be tested like never before.

In our SMT, the leadership styles differed and opinions about Covid-19 were varied. Nevertheless, as a collective, we decided to come together, carried by a common purpose.

The hard lockdown was difficult. While the education authorities pondered the reopening of schools, the buzz on social media depicted teachers as lazy. I felt disturbed and undervalued; it was difficult to bite my tongue. My response was limited to the teacher critics and especially to the Department of Education. I was warned about young leaders committing career suicide if they appear too vocal if they dare criticise their employer. The risk was too high; I had children to feed.

We, as teachers, found ourselves in a whirlwind of misunderstandings and confusions during the lockdown. The dual role of being a mother and teacher had unrealistically high expectations which I could barely meet. People would fondly make remarks, "Your children are so lucky; they have a teacher as a mother." The blessing of being at home with my children and fulfilling my duty as a teacher felt like a curse fuelled by frustration. Often, I had to choose between school preparation and spending time with my children, never mind teaching. There was a constant battle between schoolwork and my family, even greater than before. The best I could do as a teacher-mother trying to keep things together was to encourage reading for enjoyment and educational screen time, anything to keep my children occupied while I work. Multitasking became difficult and it was extremely tiring.

When the call first came to teach from home, I was excited and thought it would be fun. This enabled me to make use of all the computer skills I acquired over the years through attending CTLI workshops. Previously I found myself annoyed with the slow progress of the migration towards e-learning in the education sector. I knew this would be the time to apply my skills. I found myself creating Google Forms activities into morning hours to share with the class WhatsApp group and our newly designed virtual classroom on Google Sites. Parents left the group one by one as time went by. I could never make the link until I saw some of my learners fighting on Mitchells Plain's streets for promised food parcels on the local news. My heart was in shambles. I felt ashamed requesting evidence of completed schoolwork while my learners were fighting against poverty. Yes, I had a duty to perform, but how could I continue knowing my learners and their parents are struggling. Few weeks into the lockdown, the SMT volunteered to serve the school community by means of opening the school feeding scheme as requested by the WCED. Assisting with meals daily, knowing our learners were fed, outweighed the initial fear of being at the forefront of the battles faced.

The pressure on these parents was harsh as they did not have the resources to comply with the demands of home-schooling. In some cases, the lack of formal education was a concern as assisting their children became difficult. I simplified my lessons and included voice notes without no success as data became the next challenge. Unfortunately, there were only a few learners who had access to devices with internet connectivity. I continued with the lessons even though I did not receive notifiable responses. I was mindful of the stressors parents had. Some parents worried about schoolwork other worried about their next meal. I wanted to alleviate some of the stressors, but it felt like a catch 22 situation. Despite my uncertainties about whether I should continue WhatsApp teaching, my WhatsApp line remained open for general discussions. I was well aware of the ripple effect stress might have on my learners in their homes. At this stage, I needed my learners to be content within the context we found ourselves. I reassured the parents that I will reach for all the tricks in my hat to ensure quality education when the schools reopen.

As the South African lockdown levels changed, the teaching and learning strategies changed as well. Moving from level 5 to level 4, some restrictions were lifted, and schoolwork became accessible to learners. We, as teachers, went back to school and the parents could collect take-home packs from school. The ideal was in recording educational videos to assist the parents, but my failed attempts had me in stitches.

In the meanwhile, we anxiously welcomed the Grade 7 learners back. Previously I have done some low-key acting in church, but this was the best I have ever attempted. As I enter the school gate every morning, I inhale and exhale as I put on a brave face. In front of the learners, I would be advocating government and provincial Covid-19 protocols, simultaneously shaking in my boots. Those days were tough, to say the least. I would often drive home in a daze, thinking about how I could manage all my duties efficiently. Preparing lessons for the Grade 7s, designing supporting materials for the Grade 4 WCED lesson plans, schooling my own children at home, and at the same time fulfilling all other daily tasks. Despite such busy schedules, professional development sessions continued. We attended Microsoft Teams and Zoom meetings left, right and centre, and sometimes in the car commuting home.

Given our workload, lockdown level 3 could not come fast enough. However, teaching on the Cape Flats also meant dodging bullets, SARS-CoV-2 bullets. Children and adults made little attempt to adhere to the lockdown regulations. Children were playing in the road with no social distancing or masks in sight. Driving to school and going back home was like moving between different lockdown levels. My nerves were shot.

To remain optimistic, I studied all the Covid-19 guidelines and policies that were sent daily. Minimising the possibility of contracting the virus became an obsession. My health and the health of those around me became my personal responsibility. Eventually, with all the responsibilities on my shoulders, I experienced teacher burnout. My immune system grew weak. As I recovered from one viral infection, the next would follow. The teacher assistants arrived in time to alleviate some of the many responsibilities. I saw them as the little angels who brought great relief. I was so grateful. The relief was short-lived since our Grade 4s returned shortly after. Most of my learners returned to school on their scheduled days and I was in full-scale, formal education mode.

Teaching went well and I enjoyed spending time with smaller groups of learners. Nearing the end of the year, the WCED made a final call to learners who had not yet returned to school. At that point, I knew I had to intervene. There were some of my learners I haven't seen in months since the lockdown started. I requested home visits from the office. Previously I would never attempt this; I was too scared of the gangsters in the area. Before I knew it, I was in front of a learner's house who had otherwise complete all her school-based tests successfully. As I pulled up, I heard a voice, "Hier kom haal hulle jou" (Here they are coming to fetch you). By the looks of the surroundings, I could sense the family hardship. As the learner approached, the tears rolled down her unmasked face. The mother ran frantically towards me, still trying to get fully dressed while attempting to explain her child's absence. All I could say was, "It is fine, Ma'am, I just need her to come to school." She returned to school the next day and never again.

Despite the fear and uncertainty of pandemic teaching, there were two things I enjoyed as a teacher. Social distancing (1.5 metres) gifted us with smaller classroom sizes. The ratio of 18 learners to 1 teacher is something a government school can only dream of.

I indulged the opportunity. One-to-one teaching in these smaller classrooms worked wonders in getting the nitty-gritty concepts across to a learner. Learners were more eager to engage, and their self-confidence improved. I also found that, in these new conditions, the learners were more respectful of each other and their possessions; overall, behaviour improved so much so that detention classes were suspended.

As we approached lockdown levels 1 and 2, the social distancing requirement was reduced to 1 metre apart. Once this announcement was made, I was on the edge of my seat. I waited anxiously for an official letter to inform us we are going back to full classroom capacity. I was relieved to learn that existing safety measures remained unchanged. Slowly curriculum planning and general decision-making became less erratic.

By the fourth term of 2020, we finally reached stability in schools and classrooms. It was a growing concern that the curriculum would not be covered by the end of the year. The curriculum was 'trimmed', and yet it was difficult to complete all the topics. Mastery learning was attempted, yet I wish I had more time.

There were positive elements coming out of lockdown. As the year came to an end, I was pleasantly surprised at the increased parental support and involvement in the learners' academic work. Parents were more concerned than before about their child's progress and their ability to study for their tests. This was heart-warming even though WhatsApp messages from parents requesting assistance sometimes came at midnight.

As the year came to an end, our school was hit with its first positive coronavirus infection, and before long, we had a few more positive cases. As a school, we were back on an emotional rollercoaster as the tension in our morning devotions could be cut with a knife. Prayers went up; confidence came down. As the news broke of yet another colleague in isolation, uncomfortable silence became the order of the day. Dead stares. The virus had hit too close for comfort and I was forced into quarantine. The dreadful phone call to the school was difficult as it was time for promotion and progression. In this time, teachers should not dare stay absent due to the workload. In my mind, I created different scenarios of how this news would be perceived. The battle of the mind was extremely difficult, if not the most in this time.

In 2020, I realised the depths of being a leader and the influence you have on those around you physically and virtually. Being in an appointed leadership position was definitely challenging. Despite the fear and uncertainty, I have managed to grow as a teacher leader and strike meaningful partnership with not only teachers but other educational leaders in the sector as well. I am grateful for the lessons the pandemic brought along, but most of all, I remain grateful for the gift of life.

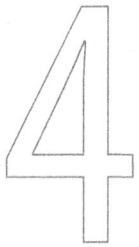

Teacher stories about pandemic teaching

4.1 Pressure

> "I felt like an incompetent teacher."

ASHEEQAH DAVIS
Simon's Town School (Western Cape)

As a novice teacher, the year 2020 was supposed to be the year of new beginnings and endless possibilities. Instead, I got restrictions and uncertainties. The lockdown had a significant impact on the education system. The curriculum needed to be 'trimmed' to salvage the lost time. In doing so, the department of education had a few expectations from schools and teachers, which then filtered down to the learners. The education department expected us to embody this 'new normal' when in fact, nothing about the situation was normal.

Three months of online learning, teaching and assessing resulted in sleepless nights and constant headaches. With the 'new normal', it was time for me as a novice teacher, as a pioneer of a new subject in South Africa – Marine Sciences – to fasten my straps and hold on tight as the pandemic wave struck.

I remember when teachers received the word from the department to continue sending work home to learners during lockdown like it was yesterday. The pressure to ensure that each learner received and understood the content became an administrative nightmare. This was not part of the plan. This was not how the year was supposed to go. I have planned so many excursions, rocky shore explorations, aquarium visits and camps. This was not in my plan at all.

During the first week of lockdown, I sent tons of work to my learners every alternate day. Eventually, I lost track of which day of the week it was, who was actually doing the work and if they understood the content. The department had expectations from us and just like we had certain expectation from the learners. Being a real-life teacher was a memory as I got caught up in the new demands. I recently dipped my toe into the education field, and I wanted more of that, not this 'new normal'. I wanted to teach in the classroom with spoken words, hand gestures, and human interaction was my comfort zone.

We had two weeks of sending notes to learners homes. The stress I felt must have been ten times worse for the learners. We were swimming in uncharted waters and I was barely keeping afloat. University training did not prepare me for teaching during a pandemic.

I needed reassurance. I needed someone to let me know that what I was doing was enough. I needed to regain my passion for teaching. I needed to know what my next step was. I kept thinking about how the education gap between the privileged and the poor was widening with each passing lockdown day. This made me angry. I was now not only angry at the virus but also angry at the state of our education system. I needed to do something about what I was feeling.

Our principal sent us online courses offered by the Cape Teaching and Leadership Institute (CTLI) that looked at different digital pedagogies. This was it, I thought. The Department was at least making some effort to provide support to teachers and bridge the gap between those two worlds in which our children learn. A trimmed curriculum was not enough. I attended more courses than I can remember. I was not only doing this for the learners but I also did it for myself. I knew that I needed to be fully prepared and equip myself to address this growing inequality in schools. I was determined to make learning interesting, fun and interactive again.

Of all the digital pedagogies encountered in the online courses, a few were appropriate for my school's context. Those were Zoom and WhatsApp Messenger. I used both facilities in my teaching and I must admit that it made a huge difference. There were some challenges beyond my control. The main problem with adopting digital pedagogies is to ensure that learners had access to data or internet connections. Most of the learners that I teach live in a hostel at Simon's Town School. They come from all parts of South Africa, including remote villages, where a signal is hard to find. Throughout my lessons, the learners would disconnect and reconnect, making teaching difficult. This disruption of online lessons was perhaps not so different from teaching in a real classroom after all.

Zoom sessions quickly became part of my daily routine. I regained my passion for teaching. I was still able to interact with my learners and use hand gestures which I love doing. The Zoom sessions are what I looked forward to each day. Having some form of human interaction was just what I needed. After all, we are highly social beings, and that is what set us apart from all the animals. I needed to accept the change, and in doing so, I found myself changing and growing at the same time.

Charles Darwin put it best, "It is not the strongest of the species that survives, nor the most intelligent that survives. It is the one that is most adaptable to change."

CHRISTINE FOURIE
Toevlug Primary School (North West)

What an experience! One can try to explain, create an image, but it is impossible to imagine what a teacher needs to endure during these trying times. The responsibilities are endless and the curriculum daunting. Skills are acquired, you adapt, you 'change'. You greet your colleague from afar, wondering whether you would see each other again the next day. You welcome the learners, but would they be safe? Would they follow your rules at home? The image of a child on a ventilator flashes through your mind. You close your eyes and say a prayer, hoping that it would be enough. Would it, though? Uncertainty hung in the air.

I am an educator working in a full-service school with 880 learners outside of the town. The language of learning and teaching at my school is English. I am a qualified mentor and assessor, a prayer ministry counsellor, with a distinction for my education degree. One can imagine that these qualifications would make it easier. It does not. Apart from the basic rules set by the government, the school also enforces health and safety rules. I have a checklist before going to class: sanitiser, my mask and shield, an extra mask for a learner (in case it gets lost/stolen/broken/wet), sanitising wipes, water bottle; wait, leave the water bottle so that I can carry my textbook, notes and a box for all the papers.

I use flashcards, pictures, videos, songs, worksheets and even puppets to encourage teaching and learning since the learners cannot see my mouth or read my lips. In reference to the latest circular, it is immediately evident that the school does not have enough classrooms or textbooks, toilets, educators, cleaners, or resources for learners with barriers or disabilities. Learners with special needs struggle to keep their masks on and to take care of the masks. They need to be continuously reminded of the rules and distance between them. The frustration builds up. There are few answers to pressing questions. Mental health, financial implications, feeding schemes, communication, and absenteeism are duly reported.

Teaching under lockdown was challenging at first, to get used to the way things need to be done and how to act in different situations. As some teachers with health risks were not at school, the other educators had to occupy their subjects and periods in the class. Without extra teachers to assist, we felt stressed, overwhelmed, and the workload was unmanageable. Educators were drained and overworked. With assistance from the management of the school, we were given motivational speeches, guidance, advice, and a small gift to boost morale. Some days there was a shoulder to cry on. We managed to do what was expected of us and even more. We could experience the satisfaction of work done and learnt how to be sensitive to educators that came back to school after testing positive for Covid-19. Though physically separated, we could be closer together socially with the use of technology.

Teaching under lockdown can be demanding, but change can be good. It takes us out of our comfort zone and allows us to develop, grow, and even change. In the classroom, I am more vigilant about the health and welfare of every learner (masks, distancing, hand sanitation). I now give more attention to cleanliness and attendance. Books are marked at the end of the week. Worksheets and notes are provided as there are not enough textbooks.

Teaching is not enough. I had the privilege of working with an inspiring committee within the school that distributed cooked meals from the school's kitchen to the learners and children of the community every day during the lockdown. Learners of all ages lined up at the school's gate hours before food would be distributed, no matter the weather. Then I ask myself whether these learners would be able to attend my online classes.

One needs to be realistic in this situation and use alternative methods of education. Worksheets with reading passages and writing exercises were also distributed at the gate. There were educational programmes on the local radio and posters on the school gate. This was quite time consuming, but when I locked the kitchen every afternoon, I felt that I needed to do more. Toiletries, school shoes and food parcels were also donated during this time.

There is a difference between teaching learners in class and at home. Home is not ideal for learning for many children. Underprivileged learners in a household with illiterate parents or even absentee parents will not be able to get access to data or devices for online classes. On the other hand, there are only 20 learners in a classroom according to regulations, and the learners can benefit from individual attention and assistance. One can even see improvement in the learners' marks and discipline. The curriculum was trimmed, and fewer assessments required. Meetings were held online, and only important information was sent via email or WhatsApp. One could get used to this way of teaching.

I did research and found that worksheets with pictures and short notes and activities would assist the learners in completing the curriculum. The teacher must also create a pacesetter to monitor the pace of teaching in the subject. I am positive that the revised curriculum will be covered by the end of 2020. It is important to do proper planning for 2021 because some topics were not addressed in the amended curriculum, and it needs to be taught.

Learners' overall academic performance is not on standard due to the lockdown, school closure due to Covid-19 cases, and even phasing in and attending school on alternative weeks. Most educators are doing their level best to close the gap and improve quality learning in the time we have left in 2020. An estimated average of 70% of the learners returned back to school after the school sent letters, phoned parents and even did house visits.

There were many positives during this difficult time. I have not been sick even though the situation was stressful. I managed to learn new methods of teaching and improve student learning. There are no longer overcrowded classrooms. I am more intact with my mental and physical health. I am more motivated to try something new, for example, writing this article. I would never dream of doing something like this a year ago.

Tania Tryon
IG Griffith Primary School (Gauteng)

The school introduced an online platform for learners on- and offsite to engage actively with teachers and continue covering content from the department's trimmed curriculum. This online platform helped to enhance the learning experience, and this made me think about how I could use my current circumstances to improve my teaching and provide much-needed academic support to my learners.

I now realise that there is a definite place for a blended learning model in schools as this can improve learner's engagement with the curriculum through the creative uses of technology. As the lockdown eased, the learners began returning to school. I decided to continue using the online platform to aid my class-based teaching. I found this to be beneficial to learners who, as the year progressed, began to enjoy the benefits of class-based teaching in conjunction with the online platform to give much-needed depth to the content in the curriculum.

The learners, however, were still experiencing feelings of stress and uncertainty. Such mixed emotions came as a result of the many underlying issues they were experiencing. Loss of employment of a parent put financial and emotional strain on households. A family member who succumbs to the coronavirus leaves an emotional void in the lives of learners. In addition to all of this, many learners were still uncertain about their high school applications. Some learners were initially accepted into high schools, which later contacted them to inform them that they would have to withdraw their provisional acceptance and reapply and begin the application process again. These children should not have to stress about such things given the kind of year they endured.

I have had countless conversations with my learners to try to unpack underlying feelings that were making it difficult to prepare and study adequately for the exams. Most learners would say that even though they were experiencing a great deal of emotional pain and loss, they would rise above their existing pain. They vowed to give their best during these exams. Despite the many challenges and obstacles of the 2020 academic year, they still thrived.

All of this has taken its toll on me. I have never worked so hard to teach children, but more importantly, to teach them well. I supported my learners to the best of my ability, often at the expense of my mental health. At the moment, I can only think about taking one step at a time and one day at a time.

Elizabeth Gouws
Berzelia Primary School (Western Cape)

Teaching under lockdown was an experience that I will never forget. As the days passed, I could not accept the fact that I must live with extra pressure, extra responsibility and that my life would change drastically to teaching with a mask, walking with a scanner and sanitising all the time.

Working in shifts with my learners decreased the contact time. However, the most challenging adjustment was the response to what will happen if and when a learner tests positive. There were specific steps to follow as a teacher, the one trusted by parents and relied on by learners. I had to be a role model for them in difficult times. I had to stay positive, extend my skills, and plan my lessons all at the same time.

I salute our department of education for their readiness and positivity in the crisis. For three terms, these officials had to adjust the curriculum for the different phases under uncertain conditions. Zoom meetings kept us on track even if we did not always understand the updated information. Internet difficulties did not help. Still, the department did not give up, for they walked this road with us.

Lastly, I can just thank God for the cooperation received from the educators as a team. We have a trimmed year with success, despite the challenges we faced during the lockdown.

Lindsay van Zyl
Greenlands Primary (Western Cape)

Not too long ago, we as teachers joked about when the coronavirus surfaced in the media. Little did we know that the virus would be the reason for the new normal in education and society.

At first, when schools had to shut down earlier than expected, I thought this was a brilliant decision made by our government. It honestly felt that our health and safety were put first. In the first week of lockdown, things went okay; I relaxed and rested, counting off the 21 days. Then reality strike as the infection numbers went up and we faced a state of emergency. I started to worry as an educator. I thought of my learners. With schools closing so fast, I did not really think of giving them extra homework.

When lockdown was extended, it made me feel worse because my kids were left with no schoolwork. I felt like an incompetent teacher. I could not shake this feeling. I started inquiring on social media platforms what other schools are doing during this time. Asking made me feel even worse since teachers were teaching via various platforms, and here I was sitting at home, wondering how I could reach out to my kids. At that moment, I felt that I had failed my learners. I had to quickly think of other ways to get them going while being at home. I realised that I just could not sit back and wait for better days. I had to make a plan.

Online teaching was not going to work where I was teaching. Parents asked why they must use their data for schoolwork while others were simply unable to afford the data cost. As a result, 'online online' never happened. A simple business WhatsApp group was the only online presence created. The sole purpose of this group was to communicate with parents. This is where I decided to hand out hard copies of work booklets for my learners. The learners were then able to complete these at home.

I had no choice but to do it old school style. This method also presented difficulties. It was hard to get hold of the parents. Some parents collected and others did not even bother to show their faces. We had different types of parents. One group moaned and groaned that the work was too much, while others requested more work.

I cannot deny the fact that this was a stressful task. At this point, all educators at the school wanted to print and copy work for their learners. Much patience was required under such pressure.

When schools reopened, the situation became worse. There were so many changes. We had to create a new and safe normal for our learners. We started by rearranging our classrooms to accommodate the lockdown rules and regulations. These changes were overwhelming at first. You had to divide your class into two and then teach the same concept twice a week; this was exhausting. If this was not enough, you had to reteach the concept for those learners who were absent and those at home with comorbidities. Teaching was strenuous for another reason: you basically have to teach the parent to teach the learner. At his point, I felt like a parrot repeating the same concepts over and over. This became our new normal, unpleasant but true.

It was and will still be difficult to cover the curriculum under these circumstances. I feel that I did not reach my goal with the curriculum, although it was trimmed. The time just did not allow me to cover everything because you are teaching only 50% of the content, which then had to be repeated. Even the trimmed curriculum could never be taught in full, given the slower pace at which learning takes place for many of my learners. I strongly feel that they will not be ready for 2021; there are too many gaps that need to be covered.

Nevertheless, as the learners and parents got used to the two-day system at my school, we noticed a remarkable improvement. More learners showed up as the lockdown levels dropped. It still did not improve teaching and learning, but it got better every day. We faced new challenges daily and yet had to protect our precious contact time. As the term went on, all of my learners eventually showed up for school. Not all of them were on the same level, and some missed out a lot due to absenteeism.

It was not all doom and gloom. Firstly, having 20 learners was only a dream, now it became a reality, but honestly, one does miss the other 20 children. Secondly, in this difficult time, I learnt that being fearless was difficult but possible. And thirdly, not once did I fall ill even as seasons changed, for which I am grateful. I now know that I am part of the frontline workers.

4.2 Pedagogy

> "The Covid teaching freestyle dance is trickier, confusing and with harsher consequences."

Brenda Shelley Jordan
Alexandra High School (Gauteng)

The air was filled with silly chatter as my Grade 12 class prepared for the first term athletics meeting. Their excitement was soon to be replaced with uncertainty. Messages were hurriedly sent to teachers to prepare work as quickly as they could. The printing room was filled with the sounds of paper being pulled along conveyor belts. It was hot off the press booklets being copied. The synchronised energies of teachers, 'admin' and ground staff heralded the storm that was to come.

As the final bell rang, the children left the building. We locked our classroom doors and hurriedly said our goodbyes. The anxiety of the unknown crept up on me. Was this the end? What if … The television became our earpiece as we awaited news from the President.

LOCKDOWN …

My mind drifted to my students. How do we teach? We were so used to whiteboards and projectors and books. Despite the many unknowns that lay ahead, I found myself gaining confidence. I am on social media; my kids know how to use technology; this would be as easy as pie. WhatsApp and the Apollo portal would be our new teaching tools. It was exhausting and frustrating at times, but we pushed on. The kids need this year.

Despite having our own families to deal with, we were on constant alert for messages from our principal, updates on our teacher chats, and the ongoing tug-of-war between the unions and the government departments, education and health. The call to return to school came even as the virus peaked; my anxiety returned. I had not been anywhere. I had never left my house, and now I must return to school amidst terrifying reports of Covid infections and deaths.

That was nothing in comparison to what we would put ourselves and our kids through – five weeks of non-stop teaching. Timetables were adjusted. My English department taught all the grades. There was no time to prepare for what lay ahead. Lesson plans, Annual Teaching Plans and then the Revised Annual Teaching Plans. Do this. No, do that. Just when you thought you had it all figured out, something new had to be implemented. We taught nine-period days. It was brutal.

We had to do screenings amid the constant smell of sanitiser and the oh so heavenly mask. The distance between my learners and me was something I could not handle. Our jobs entail interaction, moving up and down the aisles in our classroom, making funny gestures to explain things like onomatopoeia to the juniors and *The Garden of Love* to our matriculants. The pace at which we worked online as well as in the classroom was exhausting. But we soldiered on. It was about the learners, the class of 2020.

Fatigue took its toll, but I needed to be there for my learners. Teaching under lockdown is not for the faint-hearted. It tests your inner soul. It makes you question; it makes you cry, and it makes you angry. It also makes you happy at times.

It was the year that highlighted the brutal differences in terms of those who have and those who do not. A year that brought out the best in some of us, and the worst. A grim reminder of how nothing we plan is guaranteed. That life must never be taken for granted. A year that put on display the strength and resilience of teachers. We were stripped down, exposed, and yet, somehow, we are here to tell our story.

ÄNGELIQUE TRUTER
Laerskool Swartland Primary (Western Province)

I remember preparing my kids for the intense sanitation and handwashing procedures that were soon to follow. I am always finding ways to make everything in life a teachable moment. I was not prepared, however, for what was about to happen to teachers, the children, and the future of education.

School closed earlier than usual, and my heart was unsettled. I was unable to greet my kids properly, as I did not know when I would see them again. Little did I know that a little hug I offered was going to be my last hug for 2020.

Going into lockdown with students from different backgrounds was like standing in front of a mountain that had to be scaled, except that I had no experience of climbing. How do I exchange my hands-on teaching approach for teaching behind a screen? How do I make the children eager to learn from a distance? How do I make school fun with no school? I was scared and nothing I studied prepared me for this moment. Until now, I was always proud of my style of interactive teaching.

Having 32 kids in my class from different life circumstances, I had to reach each student as an individual. Some needed more motivation and more instruction, while others simply needed a parent, a haven in which to shelter. I called them daily to check if I could help with work, read them a story, or just be a shoulder to cry on. It was not easy, but I owed them that much as I was their support system. I had no knowledge of what the right way was to deal with the new challenges and needs they might be grappling with. I tried every method possible. I figured out quite quickly that the children needed personal reassurance as much as they needed to learn new concepts.

A quote by Mark Twain gave me the necessary inspiration: "The secret of getting ahead is getting started. The secret of getting started is breaking your complex, overwhelming tasks into small manageable tasks, and then starting the first one." My first task was to take care of their basic needs since one cannot build a house on a cracked foundation. I explained to them the reality of the situation, what I do to cope, and that we are all in this together. We usually laugh and play together, but we also cry and face life together. This new approach lasted for a few weeks, and soon the children would adjust to the new lockdown rules.

Given the distance between us, I still needed to get my teacher fix. I decided to meet my students halfway by joining in on social media. I followed their trends and carefully observed what made them Tick …Tok. A social media platform was the stage for new curriculum-based performances. The students, my number one fans, motivated me to keep up the singing and silly dance moves. Soon ten followers became 100, and before I knew it, I was reaching 50 000 children all over South Africa.

I engaged with my students on a level that I would never have done before. I was finally able to make them excited about learning despite the surrounding chaos. Red lights started to flash when I realised that I was unable to reach all of my students online. We like to say in our class that "we are a family"; that means nobody gets left behind. Students who were unable to join in on the social media fun came to the school's weekly 'drive-through' project. Here they would find me dressed up with posters and balloons to greet them while handing out hard copies of schoolwork to be done at home. I hoped this performance would motivate my learners and reminded them of how much fun school used to be before Covid-19.

When schools reopened, my learners were so motivated by the social media posts and drive-through activity that I had a surprising retention rate of 97%. Sadly, on return to school, a significant number of students were unable to cope. Reports reflected broken homes, little support, and the need for hands-on teaching. As a result, more of my teaching time was spent attending to broken children and doing damage control.

On reopening, terrified eyes stared at me. Faces were masked and Covid-19 protocols were enforced. It was the sweet sounds of familiar songs from the social media accounts that made frozen limbs to slowly defrost. We could not change the situation, but we could change our perspectives on it.

We were going to tackle the full curriculum. A firm commitment was required from everyone to make this a reality. My colleagues helped designed an inclusive term plan that included most of the curriculum's suggested content. It gave me joy that we did not leave any gaps in their curriculum. It was challenging for both teachers and learners.

My students, as young as they are, have a clear understanding of what the curriculum requires. We speak about the learning outcomes that we need to reach and make joint decisions on ways we could integrate different topics to maximise learning. The best decision made was to make them a part of the goal-setting. There are still some grey areas, but we are all working on our 'recap' (consolidation) strategy.

One thing I know: my little beings will become heroes. The world needs them.

Kurt Minnaar
Teacher and content creator of Dreamer Education (Western Cape)

Teaching under lockdown was like being a dancer that only focuses on choreography and suddenly has to switch to freestyle dancing in the blink of an eye. And yes, it is two completely different concepts. Choreography is structured and well planned, almost like education. You hear the track beforehand and familiarise yourself with the rhythm and beat. You have ample time to practise the carefully thought out moves to perfection. Here and there, the choreographer will add a new move but, once again, you have enough time to grasp and perfect. Freestyle dancing, on the other hand, is a completely different ball game. When you hit the dance floor, you have a few seconds to catch the beat and then start dancing. There is not much time to think and plan. You literally just have to go. And in freestyle hip hop dance competitions, you dance to a new track every round whether you like the song or not, which makes things more complex. Here and there, a track pops up that you know makes things a bit sweeter. Also, you have to come up with your own moves. The more skilled and adaptable you are, the better. It is just that: the Covid teaching freestyle dance is trickier, confusing, and with harsher consequences. Let me explain.

I have been out of the mainstream classroom for about four years. I have been doing my own thing in the education space, and towards the end of Term 1, I signed a contract at Hyacinth Primary School. My contract with the school started in the second term. At this point, teaching through a pandemic was not something that crossed my mind. I was really amped to start teaching my new Grade 5s. In my mind, I could see how *lekke* (great) things were going to play out; the class dancing and rapping the math, all of us collectively putting in the work in a fresh way. Running new math after-school programmes, experimentation on full blast, doing home visits and getting to know the area and families better. *Yoh*, reflecting on that moment still gets me excited. Plus, it would have been the first time I tested my new teaching methods and materials with the intermediate phase in a school on the Cape Flats. It does not get better than that. Like choreography, everything was planned. All I had to do was execute my dance piece and tweak it here and there.

Boom, plot twist! South Africa goes into hard freaking lockdown. Lockdown was something I never knew existed. I mean, life itself changed, and this included my dance at school. Bye-bye choreography, hello freestyle. Oh, and what made my freestyle a bit more intense was the school I found myself at. The school was declared by the DBE as dysfunctional. I expected to encounter some challenges. However, I was not expecting to be a frontline worker in a hotspot area. The school is located in Lentegeur, Mitchells Plain. In the initial lockdown, this area was declared a hotspot. It had one of the highest Covid-19 infection rates in the Western Cape. But hey, into the schools we went to do what we do best.

As a new staff member at a new school at the start of a pandemic was definitely awkward. Everything felt cold and abnormal. The way I remember schooling, we would walk enter the school via the administration building into the staffroom. This time we had to queue and wait for our turn to be screened by staff members who looked like they were working in a science laboratory with their white personal protective equipment covering their bodies from head to toe – what a sight. Thereafter, I walked straight to my classroom and kind of stayed there for most of the day. I hardly saw the staff members, besides the few that worked in my grade and those who handed out the work I had to teach. We had a few grade meetings but only one staff meeting, and for good reason.

Plus, our school does not have a hall, so we did not have a space big enough to meet as a collective while adhering to all the Covid-19 protocols. As a result, we had to meet outside, in the quad, in the freaking cold. I guess this was the plight of most 'no-fee' public schools that did not have a hall or online system in place to meet virtually. I remember looking down from my classroom window to the quad where the support staff prepared the chairs and tables for the staff meeting. I thought to myself, how crazy is this? We are inside a global pandemic, in the middle of winter, outside in the cold, and yet it is expected of us to be highly functional. At this point, I thought to myself, I must capture this moment. I grabbed my cell phone and took a picture. I just had to. As the mantra of Instagram suggests, "Take pics, or it didn't happen". The staff meeting had to go on.

The first week started great. We had so many experienced teachers, which I thought was great. We could transfer skills and collaborate to make this teaching experience work for all of us. However, I was not prepared for what came next. Things went to the next level really quickly. One moment we had all the staff members present, the next moment half of them was gone. Sixteen of our educators applied for comorbidity leave, all of which were approved. This left me with a bittersweet feeling. I was extremely happy for these educators since staying home would narrow down their chances of infection. However, this had a major impact on the remaining staff. Almost the entire school management team (SMT) had their leave approved as well. Roles and responsibilities changed in the wink of an eye. Never in my life did I think I would be at a school where half the staff were at home for almost half a year. Nevertheless, teaching began.

I am a Grade 5 class teacher, and because this group of learners was only scheduled to return to school later in the year, I had to teach Grades 6 and 7 learners. It was agreed that these colleagues would provide us, the assisting educators, with planning and resources support. This was not always the case. On numerous occasions, to the point of frustration, we did not receive the work as agreed. Sometimes on time, sometimes late and sometimes not at all. Also, the lessons were not always structured in a sensible manner, which left us to our own devices.

Using technology would have eased the pain of doing this thing we call shared teaching. However, the school was not technologically inclined and lacked the necessary infrastructure. No online teaching therefore took place. No clear guidance was given to attempt virtual learning at this stage. The closest we came to teaching online was making use of WhatsApp. And even this approach was not welcomed by all educators. As a result, we were still making use of textbooks to make our way through the changing curriculum.

Teaching different classes without prior arrangements happened frequently. There was literally zero stability in the school's teaching plan. My irritation became worse when it was expected of us as teachers to move around from one class to another. I tried to address this issue with one of the acting leaders of the school. Moving around put teachers at risk of infection. But I was a newbie. I had to know my place at the end of the day.

Every morning I would come to school refreshed and ready for the new day and its challenges. One of the challenges was the interruptions during contact teaching time. As soon as you have reached momentum in teaching, there would be a knock on the door. Notices that had to be read and signed, and then the tuck shop story. Tuck shops were not allowed to be operational during this time, so the school asked staff members to sell goodies by walking from one class to another. Just as you start to teach, another knock. This time, the feeding scheme. The feeding scheme delegate would bring the food parcels to the class while you are teaching at any given the time of day. Feeding and teaching are both necessary, so I decided to exercise patience. This is where I realised I needed to freestyle to this new track even if I did not like it.

As a song would provide a break for the dancers to catch their breath, I thought we would get a break from school during the day. We literally had no breaks. We had to supervise the learners from the time they set foot in the classroom until they went home. During break times, we had to monitor our own classes.

My teaching was now in full freestyle mode. I wanted to get back to the known. I was looking forward to the return of the Grade 5 learners. I could not wait to meet my learners for the very first time, to do my own planning, and create some sort of structure that would work for me.

Finally, five months down the line, I started to feel the rhythm to a familiar beat as the Grade 5 learners returned to school. All learners did not return instantly, but even at this point, things started to come together. The dance was familiar, and the beats remained consistent, which allowed me to teach more effectively. Kids stood outside the class; they were screened, sat down and then class began.

I will spare you the detail of the five registers we had to complete before we could actually start teaching. It was at this time that I realised why the school's Mathematics marks were so low. Some of my kids could not read, write basic sentences, or do basic operations. As a result, we had to scale down on the work that we had to cover. There was no way we could finish what was expected under the prevailing conditions. We focused on covering the core topics the department prescribed.

Finally, we hit the last chorus of the song. It was Term 4. At this point, I knew my learners a bit better and where they were academically. I turned up my lessons and knocked my freestyle dance out of the park. I was not going to allow Covid-19 to change the way

I teach forever. One of the topics we had to cover was fractions. I thought it would be cool if I teach the concept of fractions using a drone. Drones are cool, and kids love cool things, so they should fall in love with one of the most understood topics in Mathematics.

The main aim was to capture their ever-wondering attention. Once I had hooked them, the lessons became way more *lekke* (cool). I started by showing them the drone, discussing a few basic parts of it, and then flying it. The kids almost lost their marbles; they freaking loved it. Thereafter, we focused on the drones eight propellers, which we used to cover the basics of fractions. I created a dope worksheet for them to complete whereby I traced a picture of the actual drone I used in the lesson digitally. These were some of the most memorable moments I had at school, besides the staff meeting we had in the cold.

What did I learn? Keep pushing the envelope in your teaching practice. Even though I could not implement any technological solutions at school, I still equipped myself by learning to use various platforms. During this challenging time, I am managed to engage in global virtual conferences to showcase the Hip Hop education strategies I normally use in the classroom. I am a firm believer in collaborating to bring about change in our education sector. The more you engage with other like-minded individuals, the more you learn. This way, it becomes easier to adapt to new ways in which the beat may change, sometimes with immediate effect.

Ronel Sampson
E.A. Janari Primary School (Western Cape)

Amid the well wishes, bear hugs, handshaking, and the clinking of champagne flutes, I visualised the year ahead. The year 2020 was going to be my year. I had it all planned out: I was going to attend some courses at CTLI, direct a play that I have written, and then stage a concert on that play to raise funds for my school. This was going to be the best year ever!

Then came the lockdown. By the time the South African lockdown was announced, the virus was already causing havoc in Italy. Infections in our own country were on the rise. It was obvious that something drastic had to be done.

Schools were given instructions to allow learners to take textbooks home so that they could learn independently and not lose out on any work. This was a problem for two reasons: Firstly, most of the learners opted to stay home because it was the last week of school. Secondly, due to theft and vandalism, there were not enough textbooks to go around. In normal times two learners usually shared one textbook, and classes had to borrow textbooks from each other to make sure that there was enough for the one class.

In a bid to remedy the book situation, my principal sent links to educational resources on my school's WhatsApp group with the instruction to forward them to our parents. Getting hold of the parents was not easy; most parents changed their numbers and did not update it on the school's database. The parents whom I was able to reach could not access the information, even after repeated attempts. At this point, it became obvious that I would have to step in and teach the material myself.

So, on 6 April 2020, armed only with my outdated Nokia 2 and my laptop, I reported for class. I asked the parents to have their children ready by 11:00 for their first lesson – English – via WhatsApp chat. I figured that this was the easiest way as most people are on WhatsApp. Only two children were present for the class that day. I was slightly disappointed by the turnout, but I started the lesson.

I was certainly taken out of my comfort zone when presenting these classes. I had high hopes of making videos and sending it to my learners. I spent a lot of time and effort making my first – and last – video, demonstrating how to make a sandwich for the lesson on recipes. In the end, WhatsApp rejected the video because the format was incorrect. I still do not know what went wrong, but I had to adjust that lesson very quickly, making use of text, photos and voice notes. I discovered later that I could download short videos from Vidmate in order to enhance their lessons.

I also reasoned that sticking to only my own disciplines (Afrikaans Eerste Addisionele Taal and Natural Science and Technology) would be pointless. I wanted my learners to have an edge in all their subjects. Social Science was easy enough and I found the subject matter very interesting and was able to merge some of those lessons with Life Skills. Mathematics, however, was very challenging as it was never my strong suit but viewing many helpful videos on the Internet enabled me to help them with concepts that they found difficult. I discovered my learners are quite weak with multiplication tables.

Teaching via online texts differs greatly from presenting in front of my class. I consider myself a bit of an actress, and I am really in my element when I am 'performing' for my adoring fans, my learners. Having my 'dazzling' personality shine through via text was very difficult for me at first. I went ahead with the teaching, and chatting to my learners became a fun and educational activity. The number of learners increased as well as the two girls encouraged others to join.

Despite all the good things I achieved within this group, I found that a few parents had left the group a week or so after I had added them. Had I done something wrong? I gained some understanding when one parent asked to be removed from the group as she simply could not afford the data. Another granny sent me a cartoon picture which also told a story of the hardships that the parents endured during the lockdown. In the picture, an old woman and a child is standing in front of a mobile shop, staring at the little money in her hand. She thinks: "Bread or data?" I felt that. A second, more data-friendly group was opened to accommodate those parents. In this group, I simply posted the work with step-by-step instructions for the parents so that they could help their children themselves.

When schools reopened, my WhatsApp classes had to come to an end as I was called upon to teach Afrikaans to the Grade 7 classes. In the beginning, it was quite an effort to get the learners to come to school due to the fears of their parents around Covid-19. As time went by, the parents became more trusting of us and started sending their children to school. By the time the Grade 6s arrived in July, most of the Grade 7s were coming to school regularly. By that time, I had been teaching non-stop since April. I was burnt out and it was starting to show. So, when President Ramaphosa announced a four-week break on 23 July 2020, my relief knew no bounds.

As the rest of the grades started to phase in, it became more and more challenging to get the learners to adhere to the Covid-19 safety regulations. These are children that were taught to share their lunches and stationery with those who do not have and to show affection through hugs. Policing their movements and discouraging values that I was preaching to them just a few months ago made me feel like a bit of a hypocrite at times.

I felt the pressure to play catch-up with the lost curriculum. I had only recently managed to finish off Term 2 with my learners. The learners would never be able to finish the work for Terms 3 and 4 in the two months that were left of 2020. Luckily, it is not expected of us to do so.

While ATPs and homework packs were made available, I rarely used them. The kind of language used in the material for the learners went way over their heads, especially the Afrikaans packs. I simply adapted the concepts that need to be covered to my themes and content. It works much better for me and my learners. My learners managed to write their assessments, and most of them passed with flying colours. I was confident enough to know they will be able to progress to the next grade.

Despite all the challenges, there were some positive outcomes to teaching under lockdown. Smaller classes made social distancing easier to maintain. However, it also allowed me to reach the shy child who tends to disappear in the chaos created by his/her classmates. I was also able to pay more attention to children who struggle academically. I could form closer relationships with my learners, although I needed to keep my physical distance. I also learnt that distance teaching and learning at primary school level is a possibility if you really make the effort. Both my learners and I have discovered that you can learn anywhere if the discipline is there.

MISHA KAMPHER
Undisclosed school* (Western Cape)

Even experienced teachers found themselves in the strange new world of socially distanced teaching. This transition was especially difficult for Grade R teachers. When school started for the first time, all the grades in the foundation phase had to return simultaneously. The learners' attendance was poor. They were divided into two groups: Group A with 23 learners and Group B had 26 learners. We had to split another teacher's learners as she had to assist with Grade 1, where one educator was on comorbidity leave.

The situation became challenging as I did not know her learners personally, nor did I know anything about their abilities. Returning to school in a pandemic was scary for the little ones. They were too young, in their first months of school, to get used to the idea of formal schooling. Some of the learners returned with tears in their eyes and this was extremely sad because we could not hug or comfort them.

In the morning, screening and sanitising took about 40 to 45 minutes. In the beginning, it was a struggle with these little human beings. In the classroom, it was difficult to do practical activities as we knew it since we had to adhere to social distancing norms. Teaching under lockdown also came with a load of administrative duties and unpredictable due dates, all of which placed teachers under enormous pressure. At times you had to leave teaching to attend to 'admiin' demands.

In the meantime, teachers had to make adjustments in their teaching to ensure that learning took place. New knowledge and skills had to be acquired quickly. The pandemic had taken away the interactive mode for presenting lessons. Learners were now sitting alone at a table and we were talking from the front of the class. This is a very cold approach to teaching Grade R learners.

Communication was maintained with parents via WhatsApp groups. There was no online teaching. Teachers attempted to cover the necessary content within the limited time afforded to them. Unfortunately, our Grade R learners are not academically strong enough and their progress was severely affected. Our academically strong learners will become the average Grade 1 child, and all others would be at risk of failing in the next grade or even phase. It is a sad situation.

CANDICE LIVINGSTON
Cape Peninsula University of Technology (Western Cape)

To say that lockdown caught me off guard with regards to my teaching programme would not technically be true. Due to the upheaval in higher education in recent years with regards to #FeesMustFall, I have been forced to engage with a blended learning approach as we are often not sure if the campus will be shut down unexpectedly due to student protests. So, when we went into lockdown due to Covid-19, I had two responses. Oh yes! and Oh no!

My 'Oh yes!' response to the lockdown lies in the fact that I love teaching with technology and any excuse to use technology or a blended approach in my teaching really excites me. Lockdown was an opportunity for teaching with technology on steroids. Teaching online or using blended learning has never phased me. I love the new technologies and especially the 'in' it gives me with my students. Thus my 'Oh yes!' response. My 'Oh no!' response lies in the fact that I don't get to see my students. I feed off their energy and teaching face to face is my passion. I really struggled with this, and I knew I was going to have to find a way to personally engage with my students if I were to maintain my sanity. Student engagement was key to the success of this endeavour, and I quickly realised that they missed me too.

Teaching with technology is a very broad concept and its definition allows you to interpret how you will use technology for yourself. Whether it be that you integrate media tools or apps in your LMS (Learner Management System), or whether you use different types of media (social or educational), or whether you prefer synchronous or asynchronous, that is totally up to you, and I have found that by playing around with the different technologies available, I have learnt what works for me and my teaching style. It really has been an exercise in elimination. I would like to share with you what the planning of a typical online lesson looks like for me.

In the past, I have always just relied on my study guide and my introduction to my face-to-face lectures to introduce the topic and objectives in a lesson. I realised very quickly that this was not going to work in an online environment. Students need to be reminded of the focus of each lesson as I found that many of my students did not have data to access my online lessons and were feeling lost and disengaged. In order to introduce the topic of each lesson, I prepared a PowerPoint presentation, with the objectives of the lesson clearly stated. I then created an introductory FlipGrid message, where I made a short video of myself speaking about the objectives and what I expected of them. The PowerPoint and the link to the FlipGrid were then posted on the LMS and the class WhatsApp group. What I love about FlipGrid, is that it has a function where students can respond to you, also using the video feature. It is so easy to use as there is an app for your phone and students were able to open the FlipGrid and respond immediately with questions regarding the upcoming lesson. I also used this app to get feedback immediately after each lesson too. I got the students to download the FlipGrid app onto their phones, which really helped.

I also then decided that because so many of my students were struggling with data and could not attend the online classes, it was essential that I made recordings of my lessons.

At our institution, we use MS Teams to teach our online classes, but I also used a screen-capturing program called Loom to record my lessons beforehand. Loom also allows you to project your face in the bottom corner of the screen so that students can see your face while you are lecturing. This is something that most students commented on, saying that they loved it as they could see me and not just hear my disembodied voice. In order to shrink the size of the video clips, I then ran my Loom recordings through a program called Handbrake, which shrinks the video file size and makes it easier to share. I posted these on our LMS and also shared them with the class WhatsApp groups. Students were then able to watch the videos of my lessons on their phones when they were able to connect to free Wi-Fi or when they had data.

We also set up class WhatsApp groups, and students engaged with each other and myself on these groups. What I found really helpful about WhatsApp was that I was able to connect with my students personally. An email is so impersonal, but I was able to use WhatsApp to call them and check upon them. I had one-to-one meetings with students who were struggling, and I even offered lessons via WhatsApp call at one stage, as I had students who were really struggling with a difficult concept related to data analysis. I further used WhatsApp to engage with my students by having them make mind maps of concepts that they were learning about, take photographs of these mind maps and share them with the group. We would then discuss these during the lesson. I also used WhatsApp to ask questions to which the students had to respond.

These are just some of the technologies that I used to engage my students in the online environment. These technologies can be used in conjunction with an LMS if your school or university uses one, or they can be stand-alone teaching tools used in a blended approach. My greatest struggle was that I missed the personal interaction with my students at the beginning and felt that they were not engaging with me enough, but by playing around with various technologies or apps, I was able to overcome this hurdle and finally say, "I see you."

4.3 (P)reparation

"Everything I had learnt about being a teacher had changed."

CHLOÉ SENOSI
Undisclosed school* (Western Cape)

As a first-year teacher and full-time Bachelor of Education Honours student, I just stepped into the profession when Covid-19 hit our country. I had just learnt so many things about teaching and the administrative duties of a teacher. Then came the nationwide lockdown, which at first seemed like a nice break after the stresses of term one, but when it came time to return to school in May, all the things I had learnt about being a teacher had changed, and I had to adjust.

Since my Grade 3 learners were only scheduled to come back later on, my job became administrative. Since May, I made work packs for learners to collect, created WhatsApp groups to communicate with learners' parents. As a staff and a collective grade, we tried to develop a plan on how to receive learners under these new regulations set up by the Department of Education. The first two months back at school, no real teaching took place in the foundation phase. Instead, we created work packs that learners had to collect, and if they had questions, they would share it on the group, and I would guide them. This experience was relatively new to all of us, and it was interesting to see how we, as teachers had to adapt what we knew to accommodate the 'new normal'.

Since I returned to work in May, there had been many changes and instructions by the Department of Education about the way forward and what is expected of us. Weeks later, we were informed that those changes have changed, and we had to adapt accordingly. Thus, it went, things changing almost every week. Although to some it may seem frustrating to get new information every time, I understood because, as I said, this is new to all of us, and everyone, including the Department of Education, is trying to figure out the best plan for all.

The requirements put forward by the department with respect to amending the curriculum and teaching seemed tedious at first. Still, as teachers, we are always expected to adapt to our surroundings and circumstances, and this time was no different. As teachers, we wear many hats; teacher, mother/father, friend, psychologist, disciplinarian and now frontline workers in charge of educating children while keeping them safe, which, if you think about it, has really always been our job.

As someone passionate about online learning and incorporating information communication technologies (ICT) into my teaching, I was keen to teach online. However, the reality is that not all learners have access to data and devices to receive online learning content. I did a survey asking my learners parents how many of them have internet access and devices at home for learners to use, and many parents of my thirty-eight learners indicated that there is no internet access or devices at home for learners to use. This is a massive disadvantage since online learning would have allowed me to bridge the gaps in their education that formed due to the lockdown. Since online learning was out, I resorted to printing work packs and handing out work to learners at the school gate every few weeks until learners return. Another issue I encountered was that not all parents gave their numbers, and so there were learners whom I could not make contact with, and they did not get any work, pushing them to a further disadvantage.

From January 2020, learners received one full term of teaching and when lockdown hit their learning came to a halt. This disruption lasted months, and when learners finally returned to school, there were uncertainties and school was open and shut in August again. When school finally opened for real, learners were first educated on Covid-19 and safety precautions such as social distancing and washing hands. This disruption caused there to be a vast gap in learners' knowledge, the curriculum had to be amended, learners were not attending school every day, and some parents chose to let their children work from home. Learners definitely will not complete this year with all the knowledge they were expected to learn this year, and this might cause a ripple effect since next year, when they progress to the next grade, they cannot be expected to know things they did not learn this year.

Teaching under lockdown was definitely a new experience, one that I hope we never have to do again. However, if I look at the positives that came out of teaching under lockdown, I would say that due to social distancing, we had to have fewer learners in a classroom and teaching fewer learners meant I could work one-to-one with them and reach more learners. Teaching under lockdown showed me I am capable of adapting to any situation and teaching under stressful conditions. It allowed me to think creatively and out of the box to find alternative ways of educating learners.

FELICIA BAM
Curro Roodeplaat (Gauteng)

It is pouring with rain here in Tshwane after days of extreme heat. The rain brings a welcomed relief. Just as weekends away from school brings relief from having to constantly observe Covid-19 protocols. No learners to watch over and remind of not playing rough tumbling games, which the boys love and do so well. No reminding educators to remain vigilant for the sake of their colleagues and learners. No online classes. Just welcomed rest and glorious rain.

I am an educator in early childhood development (ECD). I am also a Speech and Drama teacher. My motto as an educator is and always will be *Non Scholae Sed Vitae Discimus*. I have always incorporated that into my lessons, no matter what the age group. Suddenly … I am challenged to continue believing that motto, and I am challenged to let others believe that too. You see, I am an educator at heart, but in 2020 I found myself leading a preschool with nine staff members and 75 learners through a strange new environment.

As was the case with educators everywhere, we had to adapt and fast. I work at a private school, a well-resourced and privileged institution. As we grappled with the meaning of this new normal in our individual lives, there was the realisation that our young learners were at home. They were not receiving any teaching while our clients (the parents) expected that we continue to deliver high-quality education to their little ones. As ECD practitioners, we were certainly not prepared for online teaching.

The most important adjustment we had to make was also a morally challenging one. Whereas before, we advocated for 'as little screen-time' as possible, we now had to do the complete opposite: compile and present lessons via WhatsApp, Teams and PowerPoint. What was once an occasional treat became the new standard.

Suddenly you could not just stand in front of the class and demonstrate a lesson or sit on the carpet and tell a story. You had to find a practical way to do all of that. Living alone with no one to record the lesson for you was a real challenge for one of my staff. Suddenly you had to speak louder; you had to think of material to use at home and that hopefully, the children might have at their home. We had to think out of the box. Preschool teachers generally do that well but add technology to the mix, and things become tricky.

With no audience to give a response to the typical questions you asked, you had to go solo with your speech, I mean, lessons. You could not make the lesson too long. So much data being chowed. And while I have to guide my educators through this transition, there is always that uncomfortable, niggling question in your head: "But what about those learners who do not have access to online resources?"

Our company came alongside us and sent information, tutorials, and webinars. Oh, those webinars and remote learning guidelines, endless in supply, became so useful if technology is your thing. We watched and waited and listened with bated breath to what the honourable President would say about re-opening. In the meantime, we had to continue to prepare work for the next day while juggling family, finances, and fatigue. Did I mention fatigue?

Our company remained supportive. As Head, I sent the usual inspirational note to staff and checked in with them via Teams. The last thing we wanted to do was assume that our educators were fine. Some of them faced personal challenges.

Tech-savvy educators thrived. This was their moment to shine. My shy, withdrawn staff struggled. Their lesson content was great, but they did not want to send videos with themselves out on groups. This, however, was a vital aspect of our teaching at the time and the only tangible way we could visibly stay in touch with our learners.

As days and weeks turned into months, they all became pros. They downloaded apps to enhance their teaching, they played around with ideas, and they even started collaborating. We attempted a few videos with inserts from everyone. That was eventually compiled by one educator, sent for proofreading and then finally submitted to WhatsApp broadcast groups. Time-consuming, to say the least, but the end results were good.

Quality of work would remain important despite the newness of everything. However, teaching online is not meant for little ones. They need a personal touch. They need affirmation. They need social interaction. Covid-19 came and took that away, and when our school eventually reopened, our young learners bravely adapted to all things new.

Would the parents understand what had to be done with the online content? Would the parents grasp the outcomes of each lesson? Will the parents actually do the work with the little ones? Feedback from parents often reflected their conflicted state. "I have three children. One device. Who must have access? The older sibling or the young toddler?" Often the option was for the older sibling who had to do schoolwork that was considered as *real*. Such negative feedback made us despondent, though we know this was not intended. Creating online content was time-consuming, and it just plucks away the joy when our work is not received in homes with the same enthusiasm.

We missed our kiddies. Their faces, their smiles, their frowns, their body language. The body indicators we used to gauge how our lessons are going. How would we know that what we intended for them would come across? This time around, we had to worry about learners and their parents.

Our educators had their phones, and a few had personal laptops. Our company paid for a percentage of our data usage. Still, it was more than many others have access to. Our assessments are observation-based. We do not do worksheets and workbooks. We create opportunities to learn through our teaching in and outside the classroom, and we observe.

We stayed as close as possible to the guidelines from Head Office but knew full well that online learning comes with limitations of time, content, and input. We knew that the concentration span of our young learners was very short. We knew that what we packed into three lessons per day would barely cover what we do in a week.

Once our school reopened, we quickly realised that some of our learners had regressed in areas of emotional regulation, physical development, and just general confidence levels. We spent a substantial amount of time to settle them into a new routine in a newish environment with loads of new rules, all the while comforting and nurturing the children.

We lost several learners and our baby section closed down. Young moms were not comfortable to leave their little ones at school, no matter how sanitised our environment was. Some of our parents, like many others in our country, suffered substantial financial losses.

Our company reached out to those parents as best they could. Consistent communication with our clients created some peace of mind. Parents who had to remove their children eventually brought them back. Others asked to keep their space until next year.

No matter what you do and how much SOP (standard operation procedures for Covid management) is in place, parents struggle with the decision about sending their children back to school. Some parents opted to keep their children in the safety of their own homes; others venture out in public and pray for the best outcome.

What I have witnessed first-hand in these trying times is the following: educators adapt, improvise, and overcome. I have come to learn, through webinars, a great way to grow personally with all the uncertainty around you. I have yet to convince my staff that webinars are useful. They have been 'out-teched' and would much rather sit on the carpets with demarcated blocks whilst reading stories. They would rather rotate with their smaller groups to play and learn outside.

In this time of Covid and the early learning years, I am constantly reminded of UNICEF's mandate, "no child left behind". I wish for that to become true in the early childhood development in South Africa.

SHANTA BENITHA
IR Griffith Primary School (Gauteng)

For the first time in 30 years of teaching, I was faced with conducting lessons without learners being physically present. Now virtual lessons have become the norm. Prior to the lockdown, in my teaching of Mathematics, I used technology very confidently and effectively in a classroom setting where I was present to monitor my learners' understanding of the work.

The first weeks of exclusive, virtual lessons were unsettling, frustrating, and impacted negatively on my confidence as a teacher. In addition, I had to rely heavily on resources like my own laptop, printer, scanner, and internet connectivity in planning and presenting my lessons. My approach to teaching and learning had to adapt quickly to ensure engagement with learners at a distance.

The only digital channel of communication for presenting work to the learners was the D6 Communicator application. This forum had its limitations as we were unable to have real-time interaction with the learners. With the teaching of Mathematics, it was extremely difficult to explain concepts with the given examples. I felt it was important that I explain the work verbally to my learners. I used Microsoft PowerPoint with a voice-over to overcome this hurdle. This allowed me to teach the lesson in ways similar to what I would have done in a normal class situation. Microsoft Teams became available to learners about a month into the lockdown. I then switched to using this forum for teaching. The benefit was that learners were able to contact me individually for assistance.

I realised that virtual teaching has limitations. I often use verbal communication like facial expressions, now absent, to establish if learners understood the lesson. My teaching strategy changed. I had to replace the whiteboard with an online PowerPoint presentation. It was difficult to assess if the work taught was understood, especially to my below-average learners. This was further compounded by not being able to mark books and correct errors. Individual attention could not be given to learners who needed assistance. Interaction and the personal touch with the learners were missing. This created a sense of apprehension as I could not get timeous feedback to and from my learners.

Furthermore, I was not able to encourage and motivate my learners to complete each activity. The daily consolidation of rules and bonds and tables could not be done. With virtual lessons, I do not have control over the sound and camera functions of the technology, which learners could choose to switch off.

The workload increased as I now had to teach parents the lessons as well in order for them to assist their child. Not all parents knew what was expected from the curriculum alongside uncertainty about whether they were assisting their child correctly. Those learners who had no access to online lessons also needed help. I had to reteach the virtual lessons when classes resumed. I also had to assist learners who needed concepts to be re-explained. I was forced to constantly adapt my lessons and alter my planning given the constant changes from the top.

Access was a major problem. There was no or limited access to computers and internet connections. The cost of data was prohibitive. Families, typically, have one computer which the parents use for work; as a result, learners could not attend online lessons on Microsoft Teams. Many learners missed out on key concepts discussed in those lessons. This will impact negatively on them for years to come.

With Mathematics, one concept builds on and leads to understanding of the next concept. If learners have not grasped the foundational concept, they will experience problems in subsequent activities. With the trimmed curriculum, many important and key concepts were omitted. Some of the topics were not covered at all. In essence, only about 70% of the curriculum was covered, with only about 50% of the work taught in detail.

Only about 85% of the learners initially returned to school. We had to initially make the learners feel safe. However, the limited social interaction with peers, the wearing of masks, social distancing, and new hygiene protocols impacted negatively on the learners. There was a palpable fear amongst them of infecting their parents and family members.

Pandemic teaching led me to becoming more adaptive to new educational technologies and new teaching methods. I became more digitally savvy and now feel extremely confident using these different platforms for teaching and hosting meetings. I appreciated the classroom environment and resources that are available at school. After 30 years of teaching, I never imagined that I would have to consider new ways of teaching. This has broadened my horizon and forced me to be more innovative in my teaching methods. The concept and fundamentals of teaching remain the same, but the delivery of teaching had to change. The pandemic was the catalyst.

ZJILDIAN KOOPMAN
Pinedene Primary School (Western Cape)

For schools, lockdown meant moving away from traditional methods of teaching. Online teaching was the new thing, especially after the Grade 12s returned in June 2020. The enforced changes were really challenging, like withholding physical touch, curriculum adjustments, and the low and fluctuating learner attendance.

In general, teachers should withhold any physical touch due to harassment and corporal punishment. However, I hug my kids before and after school to show love. Now, any form of physical touch was not allowed, whether between teacher to learner and from learner to learner. Sharing amongst learners was also prohibited. My learners used to take pleasure in sharing their stationery and lunch; no more. Even sharing the concrete apparatus in class brought its own challenges.

Disinfection was required following the use of any concrete apparatus, and this can be time-consuming. Teacher interventions from a distance was a challenge. For example, we were not able to stand close to learners to show them how to use the apparatus physically.

A few adjustments were made to the curriculum in the foundation phase. One of the major changes was the instruction to integrate the Life Skills themes into Home Language, and to stop doing Physical Education. Certain skills from Mathematics were left out and did not need to be covered for the year. As a grade, we structured our planning in a way where learners received take-home packages to complete on those alternate days when they were at home. However, not all learners complete their work or parents are not there to assist.

The final challenge that I experienced was learner attendance. For the winter months, a vast group of learners stayed at home when they experienced any possible symptoms of Covid-19. As a result, I could not continue with a new content area. This meant that my planning required continuous restructuring.

Being an optimistic individual, teaching under lockdown held some advantages. Class size was reduced as learners were split into two groups, each one attending school on alternate days. I taught about 20 learners a day which number increased slightly as the warmer weather came along.

Quality teaching could now take place. With the content for each subject reduced, I could now focus on teaching skills instead of trying to rush to cover the curriculum for the year. That said, the focus on skills might mean the lack of in-depth knowledge in a subject, and this will leave a gap that will be passed on to the next grade.

With the new technology, learners who used to never participate in ordinary classroom interactions now cooperate without feeling embarrassed. As a grade, we decided to divide our class into ability groups. The pace is different for each group. I can focus more on those learners who need extra attention with an area, while I could forge ahead with the other group.

Parent involvement is better than it used to be in the past. I had a rule not to give out my contact number to parents, but lockdown 'forced' me to. By interacting via WhatsApp, parents ask for assistance, and immediate feedback can be given on progress. Each teacher and learner experienced lockdown education in their own unique way. Yet, this 'new norm' of teaching will be with us for a while, and we can do little else but to adjust to these new realities for the sake of learning.

Lebogang Kekana
Pula-Difate Primary School (Gauteng)

I am Lebogang Kekana, a 23-year-old foundation phase female teacher at Pula-Difate Primary School in Mamelodi East. Teaching is a passion and a calling to me. I believe that regardless of circumstances, learning must take place. Learning is part of everyday life, and knowledge helps us make sense of the world around us. Let me illustrate.

When you go to the shop, you will check the time (Mathematics), you need to know how much you will spend, what your change will be (money, addition, subtraction) and lastly you communicate with the cashiers or people at the shops in case you need assistance (language/gestures).

Learning is vital for survival. That is why the extended lockdown (March to August 2020) was terrifying. The thoughts of keeping teaching and learning alive stayed with me. For social distancing, our learners had to be grouped and attend school according to their allocated weeks. I had two groups in my Grade 3 class which I have named: Group A and Group B.

Each group attended for a period of five consecutive days. Since I had to teach one topic in two consecutive weeks, I had to make more teaching aids and find more ways to make the lesson interesting to me first, so that the learners could also find it interesting. This was also a way to keep me sane that I do not get bored teaching the same thing for a long time.

The requirements from the Department of Education did not bother me. A good decision was to give more time to Languages and Mathematics. I am not saying that Life Skills is not important. However, when taking into consideration that learners spent the entire four months without school-based learning, it was good to allocate more time to these subject areas in order to advance their learning in these critical subjects. Even so, I made an effort to integrate Life Skills with Mathematics and Languages in most of my lesson plans.

Online learning was simply not learners in our school environment. However, I tried to reach out to the parents on WhatsApp and created a group chat for my class. In that group, I posted some activities to keep learners busy. The disadvantage was that not all parents were contactable.

Life goes on and waits for nobody. Teaching must happen. I managed to cover 62% of the curriculum for Grade 3, Term 3. Yes, the school year continued, but I knew that the remaining time would not be enough to cover the content specified in the Adjusted Annual Teaching Plans of 24 August to December 2020. Teachers in 2021 will have to bring in the knowledge of concepts from the previous grades. As a teacher, you cannot introduce a new topic to learners if they have no prior knowledge of that area.

I had 43 learners, and luckily 42 of them returned to school. Although Covid-19 came with more disadvantages than advantages, there were three positive things worth noting. Firstly, due to the reduced number of learners in a class, I was able to give learners more attention. Secondly, I could see more clearly the full potential of each learner and identify where they needed further help. Lastly, learners are now more confident to participate and engage in lessons as a result of the smaller learning groups.

4.4 Pioneers

> "Within the first six months of lockdown, my YouTube channel had gained more than 1 000 subscribers. The lessons had more than 50 000 views."

ELZANE UNGERER
Koningspikkies Preschool Centre (Western Cape)

My heart stopped for a minute when the lockdown was announced. A lot of things went through my mind: Won't I be able to see my learners? Will we be able to pay our bills? Will my learners be able to learn? When will I get to see them again? I was so scared, and all I could do was cry, which I knew would not make things better.

All around the country, teachers started to plan on ways they could help their students. For me, it was tough. We did not have any Wi-Fi or uncapped data. My husband and I then made the decision to go and stay with my parents, where there was uncapped data for me to assist my school and my learners.

I used different ways to reach my learners, such as Zoom, Microsoft Teams, WhatsApp messages, and pictures. I made lots of videos using an application, Inshot, to support my learners online. I arranged with my parents to call my learners at least once a week just to hear their voices and to ask them how they were doing.

I followed our curriculum plan for Term 2. I kept everything as it was and as easy as possible because the parents had to teach them in the way that I do. I provided them with weekly planners with themes, etc. Each week I develop a Microsoft Word document where I explained all the activities, the theme of the week, our number of the week, our letter of the week, etc. We also asked our parents to assist us with some easy assessment activities, and they had to give feedback through a Google survey.

For me as a teacher this was very difficult because my 'relaxing' time is with my learners and not being able to hear or see them every day really got to me emotionally. My Grade R learners, on the other hand, saw the lockdown as a very long holiday. They really did not understand what was going on and what the virus was all about. Some of them did not like the way their parents were teaching them, while others loved having Mom and Dad around them all day. Although the school year was disrupted, my learners handled it very well. All the parents and learners were very cooperative. We all worked together as a team to help the learners. This made it easier for us to support teaching and learning from home.

I was worried about some of my learners. The school was their safe place. They were assured of three meals a day, love, care, and a sense of belonging because at home, it was something different.

Coming to school every day, I teach every child to the best of my ability. I teach them values, to know the meaning of love and care, and to understand the world around them. I put a plaster on a bumped knee, give a hug when they are feeling down or uncertain, and ensure that all the children feel safe at all times. This is what teaching is about, but during the lockdown I was not able to do that at all.

During the lockdown, I struggled with poems for my Afrikaans learners. I just could not find anything of value. I was down in the dumps and so negative. One night when I got into the shower, words started to come out of my mouth, and it rhymed. I managed to write six poems, three in Afrikaans and three in English and posted on my Facebook page. I could not believe the positive feedback I received from my followers on Facebook.

Teachers started to use it to make learners aware of the importance of wearing a mask. They encouraged me to write more poems to create awareness about the virus.

I was super proud of myself when a primary school in Pretoria send me videos of how their learners value and recite my poems. I was happy and thankful that my poems reached so many people and teachers could use it to teach learners about Covid-19. I never thought of making money with these poems because that was not the reason why I did it.

My poems made it to the Top 12 'Poems in Lockdown' for the Afrikaans language monument in Paarl, and it was exhibited in their Green Gallery online. I was also asked to recite my poems over Gamkaland radio station in Beaufort West. The hard work and effort were worth it, and I can only thank God for this opportunity.

Each day was better. I could cope with the fact of not seeing my learners but could still help them to progress. I prayed to God every day just to let us go back and help them. As time went by our salaries decreased month by month. I started to lose hope, and then one --day, God provided and said: "July, you will be back."

Tanya Matthews
St Patrick's CBC (Northern Cape)

I am Tanya Matthews, a.k.a. "Mrs M teaches English". If I had known on Wednesday, 18 March 2020, what I know now, I would have stocked up on boxes of tissues, bottles of gin and tonic, and I would have completed a crash course in online teaching platforms. I did not. Here I am, months later, grateful that I am still standing, albeit it on wobbly legs.

Fellow teachers would perhaps recognise me. I am that experienced teacher with greying hair in the staffroom. The one who has been teaching, seemingly, forever. The one who knows where the extra loo rolls are kept, which key will unlock the cover of the electrical board when the lights trip, and the exact spot on the Xerox copier that needs to be thumped when the rollers mangle your question papers. I am the one who has her own coffee mug for the many sachets of Nescafé cappuccino consumed each day. I am a high school English teacher nearing the end of my career. I have taught without a break for well over 30 years. I come from the time of wax stencils and RISO machines. I have had my hands stained from cleaning marker pens from reusable transparencies for overhead projectors. I have had white handprints on my trousered legs as I regularly wiped the chalk dust from my fingers between classes. I wrote end-of-year marks in a 'green book' using a fountain pen. I handwrote report cards for scholars (not "learners") in standards (not "grades").

I have always loved my job. I love teenagers. I love my subject. I love being in my classroom. I thought I would cope fairly well with the challenges of teaching under lockdown. I was wrong. I have never, in all my years of teaching, been as stretched, as uncertain, as exhausted as I am now. I have never cried as much as I have in the past seven months. I have wept in the early hours of most mornings, watching tears plop onto my laptop keyboard, wondering whether I should call time on my career. But … and here is the twist … I can honestly say I have never been as fulfilled as a teacher as I am now. I have been reinvigorated. I have been reminded why I chose this career – this vocation – so many years ago.

Lockdown started with the premise that it would be temporary – a few weeks at most – and then we'd all be back in the classroom, swapping cheerful anecdotes about our enforced vacation. I would finally have time to clear out the cupboards, wash the lounge curtains, and sort out the family photo albums.

Two days before lockdown started, I was roped in to present a training seminar to our academic staff on the use of Edmodo as an online teaching platform and to show my colleagues how to create and upload recorded lessons for our students. The preparation for that teacher workshop had me working through the night … but it was fun! I sipped the G & T placed next to the laptop as I enthusiastically created a lesson to teach the teachers. It was a small taste of what was to come. Our head of school then announced that all lessons had to be recorded in advance and posted online for our students to access during scheduled lesson times. These pre-recorded lessons had to be uploaded on our school computer common drive two weeks before each scheduled lesson for 'quality control' purposes. Aghast, I did the calculation: I teach five classes in three grades (including matriculants). I would have to teach each class four times a week, for an hour at a time. That equals twenty hours of online classes. If each online lesson takes more than three hours to create … I would have to invest a minimum of sixty hours a week to create the lesson materials. The two bottles of Tanqueray in the kitchen cupboard were not going to be enough!

As the days stretched into weeks, I had to reinvent my approach to teaching. No longer could I rely on the strength of my classroom personality, the banter and personal interactions with my students to ensure that everyone was focused and learning. I had to make detailed, professional-looking and engaging video lessons that would be posted on my specially created YouTube channel, which, in a supremely unoriginal moment, I titled "Mrs M teaches English". I felt exposed. No longer would it be just 'my' children in my lessons; there would now be other folks in my virtual classroom: parents, colleagues and the general public would be able to peruse my lessons and judge me as a teacher. Never have I felt more vulnerable as an educator.

Here is the surprise. Within the first six months of lockdown, my YouTube channel had gained more than one thousand subscribers. The lessons had more than fifty thousand views. An even bigger surprise was that teachers and students from other schools started to contact me – not just from South African schools but also from places as far away as the United States, Taiwan, and Thailand. Through the YouTube channel, I have fielded questions and advised South African students, such as Raizel from Johannesburg, Zoe from Port Elizabeth and Nicole from one of the Curro schools. Teachers have sent me materials to use in my video lessons, joining me in my quest to make resources freely available to South African school students. Marie-Louise from Germiston, Shaun from Durbanville and Petro from Bloemfontein contributed some of their own resources for me to use in my online lessons.

What the heck has happened? Can it be that I, along with like-minded peers, have rediscovered the 'why' of teaching?

Preparing these online lessons and teaching remotely has demanded much of me. I have found new teaching methods but lost sleep; gained weight but shed tears. At times, I felt that I was losing my sanity. In the midst of this, I have found a supportive group of colleagues, friends and students in the invisible world that we call the web. People I do not know whom I would not recognise if they walked into the same room with me have joined me on this online journey. Who would have thought that the biggest crisis of my career would result in the most rewarding of experiences?

Retirement? Not yet! Armed with a box (or two!) of Twinsavers, a bottle (or two!) of Tanqueray and access to some pretty cool technology, I still have too much to learn – and much to give!

LIZETTE BOOYS
Teacher and founder of Wiskunde Juffie

I am a young, energetic, qualified Mathematics teacher with seven years of experience. I obtained my honours degree in 2019. With this package, one would think I had my classroom management under control. Honestly speaking, I have a hard time with discipline. Despite this one challenge, I am still proud of myself. I consider myself to be an exceptional teacher, academic and administrator. When we were asked to teach remotely, I was very excited. For the first time, I could do everything I wanted to without having to discipline a rowdy group in class.

Before the pandemic, I had just purchased myself a camera using savings from tutoring work. I bought it for recording lessons. Although I did not have all the equipment I wanted,

I was more than ready for teaching remotely compared to most teachers. Teaching under lockdown was a complete joy to me. I would go as far as to say that teaching under lockdown had changed my life.

Some of the major teaching adjustments were setting up modules, matching lesson plans, recording subject and having more regular contact with parents. I definitely had to make my teaching more graphic because we have so many visual learners. Visuals also make the lesson more interesting and captivating, which became even more important under lockdown since you had to get the learners' attention without them being present in a real classroom.

The lessons also had to be parent-friendly since many of the parents also cannot read and write. I had to make sure that the instructions were clear to see and had to send a voice note on WhatsApp explaining the instructions. Without that extra effort, many learners would have been left behind.

In order to reach all the learners, our school management team (SMT) had us design modules for each subject. Luckily, I was already a believer in the modular system and had long set up Mathematics modules for learners. I believe maths is a subject that needs practice, and so the mere act of writing notes is a waste of practice time. We had our modules ready for Mathematics.

Other than the modules, it was hard to make videos of high quality for different classes and different subjects on a daily basis. Accordingly, we changed our plan from daily interventions to weekly assistance to children at home. I think this is where learners experienced some difficulty as they had to work independently on modules for most of the time.

I enjoyed every moment of modular teaching but also encountered some challenges. On the one hand, I learnt new skills to enhance my video quality, such as editing, lighting, sound, etc., and on the other hand, data became the biggest challenge as I needed data for the editing program being used. I also streamed lessons online, uploaded lessons, and regularly made contact with parents via WhatsApp. All the data used during the lockdown accumulated to a large amount of money, as my 40-Gig contract would not last very long. Other than the data, I would say the overall experience was easy because I was tech-savvy. I was also able to assist other teachers when they had a tough time.

There is, nonetheless, a vast difference in teaching students in class as opposed to virtually. For example, teaching on YouTube was a one-man show. I was the only one speaking and was not always sure if the learners were on par with what I was saying. There was no interaction with them. In a classroom, I can read the child's body language and hear from the answers that they give me and the questions that they ask, whether they understood the work. I tried doing live broadcast videos on my Facebook page called *Wiskunde Juffie* so that I could engage with the learners. Once again, I could not reach many of my learners due to the cost of data, but I managed to reach other learners as well as teachers.

I persisted. It was not long before I reached 10 000 followers due to the demand for Mathematics assistance to children stuck at home. I wanted to perfect my craft and decided I needed more resources. I added a small whiteboard to the mix. It came with a challenge, though. Every time I wrote my notes to explain, I had to erase the board again. Sometimes when I streamed lessons, the whiteboard was flipped, and as a result, my viewers could not figure out what I was writing. Eventually, I got the hang of it.

Since we were working from home, and no one was allowed on the school premises, we had to make use of what was available. The most frequently used facility was WhatsApp. This acted as a forum where we could discuss the work given in the modules, and learners/parents could ask questions throughout the day (during office hours). I also made use of my phone for recording short videos to send to the children over WhatsApp. To upload my videos and make it available for them to view via streaming, I uploaded my math lessons onto YouTube.

After five months, my learners returned to school, and we navigated our way through all the Covid-19 protocols. In the first week, we had 70% of our learners back at school. After much encouragement, we had a full house. Teaching could continue. Funny enough, during this difficult time, more teaching took place than ever before. With the smaller classes that were required from the new Covid-19 regulations, I was able to spend extra time on the content learners were having difficulty with. Usually, we have classes of over 40 learners. With these large classes, it was easy to miss those individual learners that need extra attention. Moreover, the CAPS curriculum is so content-heavy that you move on anyway because you are required to cover everything. As a result, when learners did not master the concepts, we are required to look for marks to get the learners closer to the pass requirements.

The curriculum was adjusted, and this allowed teachers more time on different topics. There might not have been more teaching, but there was definitely more learning in 2020. With that being said, the weaker learner might have learnt something for the first time this year. That does not mean, however, that such learning will count for much as too much time was lost to cover much of the substance of even the trimmed curriculum.

As usual, the weaker learners are the ones at a huge disadvantage because they are the ones whose parents do not have cell phones to stay up to date with the content, and they are usually the ones whose parents are not academically strong enough to assist them. The 2021 academic year will be tough for these learners. They are going into the new grade without mastering much content.

In 2021, learners will most probably be expected to complete the annual systemic testing. These results would not reflect the learners and teachers' efforts of 2020. Not because learning did not take place, but because the systemic test will remain the same even though learners had only covered a portion of the curriculum content.

In conclusion, if it were not for this pandemic, I would not have grown into half the woman I am today. I am so grateful for growth and the opportunity to realise my self-worth, to learn resilience, and to enjoy family and love in abundance.

Ilonka Poole
Greenside High School (Gauteng)

Although the pandemic has altered the ways in which we live our lives, it has taken the South African educational system and turned it upside down. Despite the forceful presence of the Fourth Industrial Revolution in society, our education system was slow to respond to the affordances that technology offers teaching in the 21st century.

In January 2020, I started at Greenside High School, Johannesburg, excited to share my enthusiasm for the use of EdTech in the classroom. I was still struggling with the *how*. A connecting link between the curriculum and EdTech was missing. I knew my colleagues were apprehensive about the impending changes but seemed willing to climb aboard and ride the train with me. I was responsible for the Grade 8 Afrikaans First Additional Language planning and had three Grade 8 classes. Just as we settled down, the learners and I were thrown down the Covid rabbit hole.

I created a Google Classroom for all 178 Afrikaans learners. My colleagues were not familiar with this web-based platform, so I took it upon myself to manage the process. Admittedly, I was not sure what I was going to do. My lockdown plan was to continue teaching and assessment and have much of the work covered by the time school restarted. We started online classes. Most of our learners had access to the Internet, which did make the transition easier. However, it was essential to be sensitive to their individual circumstances, home lives and emotions.

Online teaching was all-consuming. I had to be available to my learners and parents all day. I had to develop learning artefacts. We did not digitise worksheets but tried to use EdTech wherever possible. The learning curve was steep for all of us, learners included. We also did 'check-ins' through Google Forms to get an understanding of how the learners were feeling. Although we were all in different parts of Johannesburg, the relationship between myself and my learners grew stronger. I answered their queries and contacted parents if I saw learners were not online. My relationships with my parents would also grow positively.

I had never worked so hard. The management of Google Classroom took so much time. I did not want learners to feel they were doing work which was not being seen. We initially chose the critical parts of the curriculum as a foundation to prepare them for the next year. Fortunately, there is a lot of overlap and repetition in the languages curriculum that could be discarded. For revision purposes, we started a YouTube channel and uploaded all work to Google Classroom.

We managed to cover about 60% of the curriculum. Most learners returned to class on re-opening, but the rotational system interrupted the flow of learning. One week at school and one week at home meant that during the off-week, learners 'lost' the learning feeling. I felt like I had to restart the motivation process each week. It would have been more beneficial to continue with online learning during the off week.

There was much to learn from teaching under lockdown. One example of teacher learning came from Grade 8 digital literacy. We went through a lengthy process with the learners on creating suitable profiles. Initially, learners used any name, and it was challenging to correspond with them. Throughout online learning, I concentrated on infusing digital literacy into our lessons and interactions. For example, when I corresponded with learners through the Learning Management System (LMS), I made them aware of their tone and language use.

I never realised how exhausting online classes could be. Initially, I started with five classes a day, twice a week. I was finished. I lowered my expectations and only had two or three classes and allowed for a bigger group of learners. I have yet to master teaching online classes. It appears that teachers shared the same concerns: non-attendance, non-participation, and information overload.

Some learners battled to settle down and adapt, but most of them stepped up and produced extraordinary work. We often did feedback/exit slip surveys, and learners expressed their enthusiasm for the online teaching we created, such as a game to become an Afrikaans Jedi. Learners with barriers to learning can use the affordances of technology to assist their learning path. One thing I learnt from lockdown is that schools need to be flexible about these new learning opportunities and move away from the idea that technology encourages 'cheating'.

We designed a performance-based assessment for our literature project using constructs which covered oral and transactional texts. We added in 'growth mindset' feedback principles and allowed for self-expression through the use of a choice board. Parents came to realise that a child sitting in front of a computer does not mean that work is being done. They appreciated the ongoing feedback. The grade book in the Google Classroom made parents aware of their child's day-to-day work rather than depend only on an end-of-the-term report card.

I binged on professional development during the lockdown and found the missing link in my learning design: pedagogy. These development opportunities allowed me to experiment in the online teaching environment with things like gamification and virtual Bitmoji classrooms. Also, I have now created a digital survey that my learners will complete once school starts. This will give me better insight into the resources they have available. Initially, I did not particularly appreciate WhatsApp as a communication tool and wanted to funnel everything through the LMS. I have changed my views, but one needs to be clear on the value and uses of each tool; otherwise, you spend all your time uploading to various platforms.

I learnt that you need to give 50% less work when working online. I had wrongly assumed that the learners were at home with loads of time on their hands, forgetting they have household duties, struggling with their emotions, and 11 other subjects. I had to take these realities into consideration with the demands of my own subject.

It was also important to put boundaries in place. At the start, I would answer messages at any time of the day or night, and it became overwhelming. A meaningful life skill is to respect other people's time. I started communicating start and end times.

2020 was a rollercoaster ride for teachers. Yet despite all the challenges, it was one of my best years in teaching.

Chandre Vercuil
Kleinberg Primary School (Western Cape)

Confused little faces greet goodbye as they hurry home on the last day of Term 1, a hurried end due to lockdown. They were not sure if they could give me an end-of-term goodbye hug, and neither was I. I, too, hurried off to gather and pack as many of the things that I could possibly think of in case I would have to work from home.

Two days later, there weren't the usual end-of-term traditional farewell hugs amongst staff as we too rushed off home. I was ready to teach from home if required, but I clearly did not think it through. After all, we are an impoverished 'no fees school' in the heart of Ocean View on the Cape Flats.

The minute I got home, I immediately started flooding my contact list with parents' contact numbers and finally, the Grade 5B 2020 WhatsApp group was created. I had provided my learners with a book to read and writing pieces per week for the three weeks that they were expected to be at home.

There was no structured work schedule at first, and I found myself working into the early hours of the morning while the rest of the family supported me into the night by binge-watching series after series. Honours assignments for university linked up with possible lesson ideas for my classroom. When I think back now, I cannot believe the amount of effort and energy demanded by wanting to produce content that the children would want to engage in; it was an exciting time.

School management gave no instructions to send any work to learners. What I did was based on my own initiative and seeing the amount of effort teachers at other schools were making. I did not want my learners to be left behind, so I sent them home-made instructional videos, produced with a very makeshift set-up – the back of a Perspex sign board for a whiteboard and my husband's cell phone attached to a selfie stick and strapped to a chair with some belts. I do not know if the number of new contacts sent my cell phone into shock, but three weeks into lockdown, my cell phone gave up on me. My husband had to make many sacrifices to support my mission to educate "by all means necessary".

At first, the interaction and report back from the learners were astounding. Surprisingly, more than half the class of learners received the content and worked through it; this motivated me to continue creating lessons and videos to send to them. Learners were transformed into reporters for Ocean View by creating videoed news reports; their creativity was unbelievable. I created some maths lessons, but when I discovered *Wiskunde Juffie* (innovative Maths teacher in this book), I started sending her videos instead with additional exercises. I have to give recognition where it is due; this lady inspired me so much more to just keep the interaction with my own learners going as well as to find new and different methods of delivering lessons.

I was invited to join a departmental group on WhatsApp. After I joined this group, the department started sharing their own lessons to send to learners. I stopped making my own and started sending the WCED's content. Eventually, parents started sending messages saying that their children were not coping. Parents and learners alike were feeling overwhelmed as they could not make sense of the lessons and were unable to navigate their way through the posters. This was when I noticed a change in the attitude of both parents and learners alike.

I discovered that most of my learners' parents were essential workers, so children could not make use of the phones during the day. By the time their parents got home, it was quite late, and often learners were already sleeping. I could sense the level of despondency amongst families, and I just wondered whether all the effort was even worth it. I had by then felt that I had lost my learners and that the send-home tasks had just become a 'must share' exercise instructed from higher up.

At this point, I asked my learners to participate in creating a little video, singing and dancing to the lyrics of the popular song 'Tomorrow' from the movie *Annie*. The submissions were absolutely heart-warming. They were still there, waiting and wanting to be involved and participate as part of the Grade 5B group. A short video was created, and it turned out just wonderfully. We were now feeling more hopeful and could not wait to return since a minister said that it would be soon. That hope was short-lived. We were disappointed on several occasions, only to return to classes six months later.

The decision for all teachers to teach Grade 7 while we waited for the return of our own grades brought on mixed feelings, exhaustion and anxiety. Covid-19 protocols existed on paper. Before long, learners threw social distancing out the window and were definitely not taking the pandemic seriously. As a result, when the decision was taken to close schools again in August 2020, I was relieved and could finally spend some time with my own two babies.

Reflecting on 2020, I could easily believe that I wasted so much time planning and creating unnecessary lessons. I could believe that this time could have been better spent with my family or putting more effort into my own studies. However, when analysing the assessments of Term 3, I can clearly see that there are some learners who have benefitted from the lessons that were sent. Those learners who were engaging in the content on their own at home had a huge learning advantage over those who did not.

It is still difficult for teachers as we try to make sense of all the information which is still being shared daily. The future looks bleak for the learners, given all the time lost, but I choose to remain optimistic. This pandemic has caused many teachers to step out of their comfort zones which lead to the discovery of strengths we never realised we had. Teachers have proven to be resilient, and therefore we will find new and innovative strategies to teach in the 'new normal' environment. In the face of a pandemic, a teacher will teach. It's what we do. It's who we are.

SHIHAAM BEUKES-DIAZ
Yellowwood Primary School (Western Cape)

Lockdown was proclaimed, and all I thought about was my school family – how I would miss seeing them for 21 days. I felt guilty. I knew that my circumstances would allow me to be isolated in my safe, loving home. Some of my learners might not have loving homes or a warm bed. Some would not have enough food to eat. For such children, school is their only haven.

During the initial stages of lockdown, I was quite eager to test the idea of teaching via online platforms. At least 60% of my learners' parents and guardians were a part of my class WhatsApp group. I pushed my own limits and stepped out of my comfort zone to create videos of concepts that were to be taught in class. I would close my room door and record for at least one hour, deleting when I misspoke and editing anything that was less than perfect, only to produce videos that were five minutes long. I expected my learners to understand new concepts without any practical activities. I would later find that only a small fraction of learners attempted to work at home. It was frustrating.

I remember videos doing rounds on the news and social media. Members of the community where I teach were outraged. They claimed that if the virus did not kill them, hunger would. The guilt crept up on me once more. I was so used to having access to 'basic' internet and social media platforms. For some parents and guardians, downloading a five-minute video would require a trip to the shop every other day to purchase data. At the end of the day, it boiled down to using their last change to eat or help their child learn.

Teaching 'online' was dreadful. I became despondent. I used to teach a class with 38 eager eyes and ears, always ready and excited to learn. Teaching a handful of learners with the use of videos via WhatsApp was not normal. I heard my voice on the video, but no reactions when I made jokes. There was no Michael to laugh loudly and tell me that I was funny. No Jamie to jump out of her seat and tell me that she knows the answer. I felt alone. I knew that my learners felt the same. I wanted to be back in my classroom. I wanted to see my learners.

The 24th of August 2020 could not come soon enough. I divided my learners into two groups to attend school on alternate days for social distancing. It had been five months since I had seen my learners. I remember walking towards my classroom that Monday morning. I saw some of my learners standing in a line, with masks on their faces. Their smiles were evident in their eyes as I walked towards them. I could not hug them, but their smiles touched my hearts.

To my delight, my learners were more eager to learn than ever before. I felt on top of the world as we discussed new topics and learnt new things. I was teaching again but also learning from all of them. They were resilient. As an adult, I had given up hope so many times during this pandemic, yet they soldiered on and through it all at such young ages. I got so carried away with certain topics. I tried to do as many practical lessons as possible until assessments crept up on me. I then found myself overwhelmed with work. I was feeding work to my learners at an unfair pace. I felt exhausted, having to repeat my lessons every other day.

Even though I managed to complete all assessments on time, I still felt that I could have used more teaching time to equip my learners for their tests even better. I was lucky enough to be able to have 99% of my learners back at school, with only one learner signed up for distance learning. Many of them performed to their usual standards, whereas a handful of learners, sadly, suffered negatively with such a huge loss of contact time.

As if teaching was not already difficult enough, this pandemic added more guilt, stress and anxiety to the basket. I fear that the last term will have an even greater negative impact on teaching and learning. The last term only had a few weeks available for thorough teaching and learning before assessments started; the curriculum had to be condensed once more.

All the negatives aside, the lockdown opened a wide range of opportunities for educators. I have found that many of my colleagues ventured into writing and even creating social media platforms to share free tips, tools and resources for educators who are not as technologically inclined as the rest. It brought me immense joy to see educators assisting and supporting one another, especially for new educators who only had one real term of teaching since they had graduated.

I took it upon myself to create my own small business in the eye of the Covid-19 storm. I knew that educators, novice and experienced, do not always have the time to create beautiful learning environments. It is simply too time-consuming, too expensive or requires a touch of creativity that many do not possess. I decided to create themed poster packages for teachers to purchase and display to make their classrooms more inviting for learners, especially during such dull and depressing times in our world. I managed to express my deep love for arts through my profession and share it with all who are willing to pay a small price.

Being "under lockdown", ironically, has uplifted me spiritually, physically, mentally, and emotionally. I have learnt to be more grateful for the little things that I took advantage of so many times in the past. I learnt to appreciate every single learner, colleague, family member and friend for who they are. Where many people have been placed on 'short time' and ultimately lost their jobs, I had been able to start a business during a global pandemic whilst still maintaining my full-time career.

I am grateful to be an educator. Every day I get to teach, learn from, and inspire young, brilliant minds. Even under lockdown conditions, I would choose teaching over and over again.

Winston Cadman
Curro Sitari & Ronnie Samaai Music Education Project (Western Cape)

I was never ready for the challenges that teaching under lockdown imposed on teachers. Initially, I was quite excited to work from home and be within a few metres from the kettle and all the other benefits that teaching from home entails. Truth be told, there are some days where nothing about this noble profession makes one happy about leaving the confines of the home or the warmth of your cat's body on your lap, especially in the winter months.

I am a music teacher (cello) and not an academic teacher. I see most of my students one-to-one in one of seven teaching studios at school, except in the cases of the school rock band, the orchestra and a couple of small group classes. So, that could almost imply that I would have it easier teaching one-to-one online, right? Wrong.

Within a week, I was longing to be back at school. I missed being in the hustle and bustle of the music department where the sounds of pianos, violins, guitars, saxophones, etc., would travel to my studio along with the inspiring voices of my colleagues motivating the students along.

I soon realised that teaching from home is terribly lonely. A former colleague once remarked that there are two things in life equally eerily quiet: a graveyard and a school once all the students have left. Teaching without children present is like teaching in a vacuum; you have to dig deep to find the creativity of the moment. Online teaching is particularly draining because of the lack of an educational atmosphere, and I soon found myself wanting to make a cup of coffee after every lesson.

Truth is, the further a student was scheduled in my day, the less chance he or she would have to see me at my most creative. I realised the unfairness of this reality and did my best to approach each lesson with the same rigour. I worked hard to motivate and inspire my music students to the extent that my teaching would guarantee diligent practising throughout the week. Those were really hopeful thoughts at the time.

Music teaching is a highly interactive activity. A teacher has to be physically and mentally invested in the process. It is about showing the student what you want to hear, especially once all the notes are learnt, and it is time to focus more on the interpretation of the piece. You cannot just talk about a crescendo, staccato, or Mozart's nimble touch on the phrases that go upward, or the emotional heaviness of Beethoven's music without demonstrating it yourself. As a cello teacher that becomes increasingly difficult because so much of the students' posture and technique determines their level of interpretation.

I realised that within a 40-minute online lesson, I would be wasting valuable time talking about posture and correcting technique over the airwaves since too much talk anyway goes over the students' heads. I decided to focus on having them learn as many of the notes as possible and hoped that there would be an end to lockdown soon. Little did I know at the time that our music department would only open after six months of lockdown.

Now that I am back at work, I have a whole lot of correction to do on technique and interpretation that makes me at times feel like an adjudicator at Idols SA or a Simon Cowell when the students look at me with that daring but unspoken question: "Can YOU do all these things you're asking of me?"

Then, of course, there is the myriad of challenges with issues like network connection problems, especially on days we had horrible weather; devices that did not always work properly, devices running out of battery power, Zoom or Microsoft Teams issues, etc.

At times, students would be late for the scheduled meeting. I would call on Teams, and the ringtone would drive me nuts … pum pum, pum pum pum pum pum!!

Eventually, I started to have fun and played along with the ringtone. I did some improvisation on the cello with that ringtone and had the greatest time when my students would answer. Sometimes they would appear upside down on their screens or some other thing that I would have to guide them with to sort out before we could start.

But the biggest challenge for me was acoustics.

At home, I have a tiny little teaching studio with terrible acoustics that sometimes drives me to practise in the bathroom or kitchen. Mostly the students would be in their bedrooms because Mom or Dad was working from the lounge. Bedrooms are notorious for bad acoustics because of carpets, bedding, curtains, maybe piles of clothes thrown into a corner or that one chair that has five jerseys hanging from it. Couple the bad acoustics from both the teaching venues with the sound coming from the computer, then that is another reason to have another cup of coffee after each lesson.

At school, however, I try to keep my studio sparsely furnished, and I simply refuse to put a carpet in there to make it look more "homely", as the Head of Music suggested I do.

No, I love the way the sound bounces back from the empty walls and tiled floor and the lovely 'reverb' I have in there.

Teaching under lockdown was not all negative.

There was Michael. Michael is a teenager who has been with me for five years. I had him from the time he was a beginner cellist up to where he is today, being able to play all three movements from a cello concertino fluently and flawlessly – and he did all of that under remote teaching during the lockdown. The difference with Michael is that he is a student of a music project that I work at on Saturdays, which is an NPO where staff members are not paid. It is purely voluntary work. I figured that if I am going to sacrifice five hours of my Saturday morning every week to teach for the love of music, then I might just as well give it my all, and my all really includes all the theatrics that goes with good teaching.

Michael is used to me making big gestures with my arms with coffee sometimes flying out of my cup as I try to teach a musical concept. He is used to me getting on a chair or table and singing his melody lines out loud along with his playing to have him understand exactly where his playing should be going musically.

Michael is a shy, withdrawn type of boy. I wanted to break down his defences and lure him into a world where the music starts to communicate with you. There was this one time I had him stand on a chair to sing his parts with me, and he did so half-heartedly; then, in an effort to get back onto the floor with the awkward limbs of a teenager, he stepped on his cello and broke the cellos' bridge in half. I had to take it home and fit on an extra bridge (do not tell my boss).

The point is, through all the years of Michael being exposed to my unconventional teaching style, he had a lot to draw from during lockdown and got that from the comfort and security of his home. He blossomed during the lockdown and finished all three movements of his concertino with musicianship that astounded me.

We finally restarted live lessons at the Saturday music project where Michael is my student. I told him to bring his laptop, and I will bring mine. We will sit in the same room but, this time, we will have virtual lessons because I got the most out of online teaching with him.

Janine Cloete
Greenfield Girls Primary School (Western Cape)

Teaching in the Time of Corona –

> It was the best of times, it was the worst of times, it was the age of wisdom, it was the age of foolishness, it was the epoch of belief, it was the epoch of incredulity, it was the season of light, it was the season of darkness, it was the spring of hope, it was the winter of despair.

While many will recognise this as the opening line of Dickens' *A Tale of Two Cities*, it would be equally fitting for a prologue when writing a book about teaching during lockdown.

Most of my Grade 6s were fortunate enough to have access to both devices and data. I decided to hit the ground running from the original return date of 1 April as I wanted to test the waters before guiding my intermediate and senior phase through the waters. We are all quite tech-savvy, with three-quarters of us being certified Google Level 1 Educators.

Whilst I do teach at a privileged school, not every child has data or devices. There were challenges such as parents needing the devices for work or being limited to one laptop for the children of the house. All these things needed to be considered and caused great distress. Every laptop or operating system is not the same, and this caused lots of confusion too.

Some children would log on an hour beforehand, while others cruised in ten or fifteen minutes later. Some would be ready and focused, while others would turn the camera off and bunk (yes – online!). I had to give lots of pep talks to encourage the girls to keep going and to keep trying, despite the challenges of learning online.

I would be lying if I claimed to have been brilliant at generating suitable and exciting content from the get-go. Man, did I fumble and create confusion as well! I would be feeling rather smug and post a task in Google Classroom with an exciting flourish only to have a twelve-year-old pointing out a glaring mistake or missing link. Mortified, I would then send off another apologetic email and have the same gaffe pointed out to me a few more times. It was exhausting!

One of the biggest challenges I faced is that we all did non-stop communication. It was very difficult to switch my brain off after hours. As a matter of fact, there was no after hours. At first, I would reply to emails/messaging as soon as I could, but then I put boundaries in place. Those boundaries, however, were knocked over like the lightest of feathers. One particular message that had me cry tears of frustration was from a pupil who sent me a mail at ten at night asking me to "reply ASAP".

On the positive side, I learnt so much during the two months we worked from home. Big publishing companies granted free access to online textbooks and teaching material. Teachers from all around the globe shared their content and spoke openly about the challenges they faced. I was filming experiments in my kitchen and editing videos: skills I hadn't really tried before. I turned my PowerPoint presentations into movie clips so that my learners could watch them at their own pace (something they told me they really enjoyed). I tried out apps like Kahoot and Jamboard. To say I came alive because I was learning new skills is an understatement.

And then there was Zoom … the meetings, the lessons, the Sunday afternoon Family Quiz (great fun). It was amazing and so wonderful to use. I don't miss it at all. In the end, it was hard work. I'm not one to shy away from hard work, but this was off-piste. I *did* complicate things for myself by trying to do too many things that I saw, especially on Instagram. Many hours were spent checking out content from teachers around the globe. There was a glut of information on the Internet, and I needed to make an effort not to go down the rabbit hole of Instagram, Facebook and the rest.

At three o'clock one chilly April morning, I found myself looking for something interesting on Marco Polo and ended up accidentally spending R1 200 subscribing to an American education website. It was then that I made a note to myself to not go overboard and to preserve the small bit of sanity I had left. I had learnt a very expensive lesson! Fortunately, the money was refunded to me a few weeks later!

I taught online every second day for up to two hours at a time. I tried different permutations, such as teaching small groups (worked well, but time-consuming) and the entire class (not the greatest). I felt like a comedian on stage without an audience. I feed off the vibe of my live audience, and their interaction with me was stilted. Many of them were reluctant to ask questions during lessons and would mail me afterwards. This was exacerbated by the four different platforms through which they were messaging me: email, WhatsApp, Hangouts and Classroom. I was overwhelmed.

There were many moments of great joy and excitement, such as when I made movies, and the girls applauded my efforts, and when we were online on the 4th of May (aka Star Wars Day), and I had a stormtrooper in my class. The videos some of my kids made of their rendition of 'Juffrou, Ek Mis Jou' by poet Jaco Jacobs was delightful and showed out-of-the-box thinking. We were at our most creative, and we came alive!

Grade 6s returned to school in June, and I was dead set against it. I felt that we could carry on online, as exhausting and frustrating as it was. Returning to school in the midst of the pandemic was ridiculous! There were clear differences of opinion as to whether we should reopen, with parents on both sides of the argument. Observing it all unfold on social media was not good for my mental health. I made myself a promise not to engage with Facebook posts that addressed the reopening of South African schools. I broke that promise many times.

To cut a long story short: returning to school, albeit at 50% capacity, was the best thing for my brave band of pre-teens. They loved the live show for different reasons. They commented that they missed the spontaneity of the classroom, the immediate help they received and, most importantly, their friends. A number of them said that they spent too much time online, and they had device fatigue. Parents commented in those first days back that they dropped off anxious daughters and picked up happy girls. They could no longer claim that they had submitted tasks or hadn't received emails and they soon caught up.

One unfortunate aspect of online teaching was that there were girls who slipped through the cracks whilst working from home. They either couldn't come online at the scheduled time, or they didn't take to it as well as their peers did. Parental support wasn't always available, even though I tried my utmost to give work that could be done independently.

Online learning requires great self-discipline, and not every child could manage that either. Even upon returning to school, these children would battle to complete work on their work-from-home day.

2020 was a bizarre year in teaching. I learnt so much in terms of technology, but mostly about myself. Having taught at a disadvantaged school for 15 years, I was extremely aware of the privilege I enjoy as a teacher in the leafy, green suburbs, and I ran the gamut of emotions from anger (at the previous and present governments), frustration with the national and provincial departments of education, guilt about my and my class' access to teaching and learning, and the overwhelming demands placed on teachers during this period. I found comfort in the fact that teachers around the world were in the same storm, just in different boats.

The learners at my school were ready for 2021. Most of us managed to cover the revised curriculum thoroughly, and the girls will be able to cope with the demands of the next grade. How they will cope can only be gauged as we go along.

In 2020, I felt like a web browser with 30 tabs open at any given time, but I still found time to bake banana bread!

Gary Hendricks
Uitenhage High (Eastern Cape)

Returning to school at the peak of the pandemic, most teachers and parents had doubts and feared the worst. In hindsight, it was probably a good decision to reopen schools to continue with teaching and learning. Ironically, this was the most enjoyable and least stressful teaching experience of my career because of the smaller groups and the rotational timetable we followed. During this time, we also prepared and copied notes and worksheets for the other grades. We made use of our school bus to deliver the materials to different pick-up points all over Uitenhage. Parents and learners appreciated this effort because most of our learners do not have smartphones and access to data.

Covid-19 fast-tracked the future because suddenly, teachers who had never used technology were forced to use it in their lessons. Here I think of one of my colleagues. Like many other teachers, she did not make much use of technology in her lessons, but because she had to move between two classes, she found PowerPoint lessons to be convenient.

I was also the only Mathematics teacher who could teach up to Grade 12 level at our school. My goal was always to mentor my colleague over the next few years. Because of Covid, she was forced to take half of my classes and gain the necessary experience to teach Grade 12 Mathematics in 2021. We were also exposed to Zoom, Microsoft Teams meetings, webinars, etc.; things I am sure we would not have experienced were it not for Covid. We could even live stream our valedictory and awards ceremony on Facebook. This was amazing because all the learners and parents could also be part of this prestigious event. Now we are incorporating these technological conveniences into all our future events.

Our school also took part in the worldwide *Jerusalema* dance challenge where learners, teachers, nurses and members of the police force joined in dancing to this hit song by South African musician Master KG. The long-awaited school website was also established during this time, mainly because of the extra time we had available. Under normal circumstances, it would have taken us another year or two to get the website off the ground.

Many of the parents of our learners also lost their jobs, leaving many households without an income. A colleague started an initiative where she approached people on social media to donate money for food parcels to assist some of our needy learners and families. Our staff, former learners and teachers, and friends of our school supported this initiative so well that about 60 households benefitted from food parcels worth R350 each. We also raised funds and got a sponsorship to run a soup kitchen for our matriculants when they returned to school.

A former learner of our school was stranded in Lima, Peru, because of the worldwide lockdown. She had a return ticket to South Africa, but due to the lockdown, she was unable to use it. She, therefore, needed about R40 000 to fly from Lima via Sao Paulo in Brazil to Johannesburg. As a community, we managed to raise R40 000 within three weeks to make her safe return possible. People from Uitenhage, Port Elizabeth, all over South Africa and abroad supported this initiative.

On a personal note, the pandemic affected me financially. As a Mathematics facilitator in the Engen Maths & Science School (EMSS), I lost out on the extra income. The lockdown regulations meant that we could not continue with the programme on Saturdays. It taught me to manage my finances more effectively and to get by with what I had.

As a school, we also had to close about three times because of Covid positive cases amongst staff and learners. The school has not reported any deaths because of the pandemic. I am grateful.

4.5 Poverty

> "The reality where I teach is that children come from social and economic contexts where having food on the table ranks higher than buying data."

EMMA SMIT
An Independent NPO* (Western Cape)

I remember the first day our school received the news about Covid-19. Just a few days earlier, we were discussing the disease in our lift club on the way to school, saying, "It will never come close to us." Before we knew it, it had hit our little town. I recall a real wave of uncertainty coming over our community.

I teach at a small independent school with learners from disadvantaged backgrounds. I remember reading in the news that most South Africans cannot self-isolate because of their housing situations, such as sharing a one-bedroom house with several people. Most of my learners are those South Africans. We work in a community in which wearing masks, social distancing and owning multiple tubes of hand sanitiser is not regarded as necessary.

During the lockdown, we received regular reports of large social gatherings in the streets till long past curfew. Some of my learners were sent to stay with family in the Eastern Cape, with no form of communication available. Reaching them during lockdown was impossible, and I felt both fear and concern for my learners.

During the lockdown, people often asked me, "How is online teaching going? Do you also use Google Classroom or Zoom?" During the first few days of lockdown, I remember how eager I was. I made videos of reading stories to my learners and doing practical Mathematics and language lessons. I enjoyed the challenge of thinking about what resources my learners would have available at home and then using similar things to record activities and sending it to them via WhatsApp. However, reality quickly set in. Messages did not go through; parents started phoning and sending SMSs to say they did not have enough data or only had data after midnight. Some parents, lacking formal schooling themselves, struggled to complete the activities with their children or created more uncertainty for the child. WhatsApp was no longer an option.

I remember feeling lost and overwhelmed. Seeing how my university friends use Google Classroom, Zoom, and other platforms to teach their learners once again shed light on how my learners face many more challenges to reach academic success. Covid-19 has forced us to acknowledge the educational inequality in our country. Learners from disadvantaged backgrounds already faced challenges before Covid-19 with overcrowded classrooms, a lack of quality education and a lack of resources. Lockdown magnified these inequalities in that wealthier learners could continue with their schooling through online platforms while less fortunate learners could not.

I remember our first day back at work. Everyone stood metres apart, too afraid to be close. We were asked to wear overalls over our clothes in case someone with Covid-19 had sneezed on or touched you. Buckets with disinfectant, cleaning cloths and hand sanitiser were distributed. Colourful markers were painted throughout the school to assist with social distancing. Sanitisation stations stood outside each classroom. My 37 m² class suddenly had to accommodate 50% of my learners with a metre distance in between. The 'new normal' was in full swing.

At the beginning of June, we opened our doors to our learners for the first time since lockdown was announced. We were all uncertain and anxious that first day. Even though everything was in place, we were scared. I remember seeing all the teachers in their white overalls and masks. The learners were lining up outside of school. No students in history had ever been as well-behaved as our first group of learners. Suddenly, as the first learner entered the school, it was like all the fear just melted away.

The learners came back to school with energy and determination. Our building was once more filled with laughter and the exciting sounds of learning. It is incredible how resilient young learners can be. As adults, we sometimes expect them to become overwhelmed with their emotions and not be able to handle change. They prove us wrong time and time again.

The day we could start teaching in person again, I was so happy. Not being able to reach most of my learners during lockdown, and thus not being able to teach them, was extremely difficult. Our school is not only there for learning; it is also where most of our learners get their breakfast and lunch and the only consistently safe place they can rely on.

The academic impact of this year will only be felt in years to come. With every new school year, we as educators have certain expectations of learners. Certain concepts and skills are considered as guaranteed. However, we will need to adjust our expectations. Seeing learners only twice a week has caused valuable teaching time and consolidation to have gone lost. Due to our limited teaching time, our work pace had to increase dramatically. Learners had to master a concept much faster and for some of those struggling, this challenge was a bridge too far. I had learners who missed a whole term because their parents did not feel comfortable sending them back. Those learners still had no access to online platforms, and the academic gap they are experiencing now will continue to require serious intervention and support in the future.

The Department's decision to progress all learners to the next grade and prohibiting learners from repeating a grade in 2021 does cause some concern for me as an educator. Some learners will now be entering a new grade or a new phase without having mastered the previous one. Educators will be facing greater challenges than before.

In the "new normal", our whole approach to teaching had to change. As foundation phase educators, we could no longer follow our usual routine of reading in small groups on the carpet, doing small group practical Mathematics lessons with concrete apparatus, or physically demonstrating skills with learners. In other words, we leave learners without practical opportunities for discovery and learning. These restrictions required us to think outside the box. I decided to create a set of practical resources for each learner, so even though we could not do practical activities in small groups, we could do them as a whole class lesson so that learners could still experience concepts practically.

The staggered integration of learners brought new opportunities. Having only 50% of learners on a day provided us with a valuable opportunity to give learners the one-to-one support and attention they deserve. I realised the positive impact the smaller class sizes had when completing reports at the end of the term. I was able to provide detailed feedback and truly knew each learner, their strengths, and the educational challenges they were facing.

When we are faced with larger classroom sizes, even though we do not want to admit this, the middle group tends to get lost. We focus on strong learners because they themselves demand attention and stimulation. We also focus on the weaker learners because we are concerned and are required to provide the necessary proof of intervention. But for the first time, in a classroom of 12 learners, each learner could be seen, supported and enriched. Yes, we lost a lot of teaching time and only covered about half of our curriculum this year. But is that such a bad thing? Isn't it better to cover less, but cover it more in-depth and provide learners with more individual support?

Next year educators will face a new challenge, but with an opportunity to collaborate. We will have to attempt to cover the lost curriculum, as well as our own grade's content. Teachers must turn to the previous grade colleagues and work together. This is a time for educators to rely on one another and share knowledge. Covid-19 and the 2020 academic year turned even the most experienced of teachers into novices.

No educator could have predicted what the pandemic year of 200 held in store for us. We were forced to take a critical look at the education system and the curriculum. My wish for South Africa is that our Department of Education will take what Covid-19 has taught us to improve the curriculum and give all learners access to quality education.

LESEGO MAFOKO
Lesego Primary Public School* (North West)

My name is Lesego Felicity Mafoko. I am an educator at Lesego Primary Public School* in Potchefstroom. I teach Mathematics and Natural Sciences and Technology. The first school term was shortened with no warning. The teachers and learners in my surroundings loved the sound of the school holidays being closer than planned. It was not long before it hit me; I had not finished the Term 1 prescribed curriculum and was planning to use the remaining days to do consolidation. At this point, I realised that there was nothing I could do with regard to the content not covered for the term.

Covid-19 was something unprecedented. We had no knowledge of this virus that caused a worldwide crisis. I had never heard of whole countries going into lockdown. At the same time, we were learning new things and new terminology: pandemics, coronavirus, herd immunity, lockdown levels, etc. We had to adjust to this new normal, which required wearing masks in uncomfortable heat.

At first, I enjoyed the new normal. We stayed at home, enjoying the longest holiday I had ever had in my life. The break was good, but then I started to worry about my learners who were not engaging with the curriculum during the long lockdown. I felt compelled to do something.

I suggested in our school WhatsApp group that we use the information in our school's database to open WhatsApp groups for our learners. Through this, we could reach our learners to share information and activities. Then we realised that we would not be able to most of our learners because so many are disadvantaged. We therefore abandoned the idea for it we could not reach all of our learners, it was not good enough to only serve some of them.

Schools re-opened for the staff one week before the Grade 7 learners were expected to arrive. At this time, I fell ill, suffering from panic attacks. I was booked off for one week. I could not stop thinking about whether or not I would be able to catch up with the demands of the curriculum. I recovered, but the following week my body gave in again. My legs could not move. The doctor diagnosed panic attacks once again. Despite my fear and anxiety, God showed His mercy. I made a full recovery and welcomed positive energy and an unstoppable drive to teach my learners.

I took every day in my stride. We had time to cover most of the required topics in the trimmed curriculum. It was not necessary to repeat lessons to different class groups because they could all fit into the school hall.

As the term commenced, we managed to get 80% of our learners back at school. We reached out to the learners who did not return, especially those who had been sick before the lockdown. We communicated with these learners through WhatsApp. Learner activities were shared; however, the parents' response to these initiatives were not favourable. Teachers, on the other hand, felt that providing daily work at school and on WhatsApp increased their daily tasks tremendously. These are just some of the challenges we have encountered.

Various adjustments had to be made. I found myself being much more patient with the learners. Understandably, they had been at home for an extended time, with little to no active learning taking place. I therefore had to be patient with them. Once more learners started to return to school, the alternate teaching days became draining. I had to repeat each lesson four times to the different groups in the grade.

I am thankful for the trimmed curriculum. The guidance given helped tremendously. At this stage, I doubt whether the trimmed curriculum would be covered given the short time available and the alternate teaching days. In Grade 6 Mathematics, I found it difficult to teach mastery of concepts because our learners in the townships have already told themselves that the subject is difficult. I spend most of my teaching time repeating a single concept until they understood.

Grade 6 is the sunset of the intermediate phased and the new dawn to the senior phase. Learners must be prepared for the new phase and some concepts are new to them. The transition to the new phase was not as smooth as in previous years. I permitted learners to request assistance on WhatsApp if they did not understand the content. That was as much as one could do at the time.

Dillon Henwood
Elnor Primary School (Western Cape)

The nationwide lockdown painted a devastatingly vivid picture of the deep-rooted disparities and inequalities which are embedded in South Africa's education system. The plethora of challenges which the lockdown presented in the education sector impacted most severely on learners and teachers from disenfranchised communities.

As a Grade 5 educator at a no-fee public school situated in the impecunious, gangster-driven community of Elsies River, I was completely overcome by the exhaustive, unrealistic expectations to keep my learners intellectually stimulated. Successfully engaging my learners for nineteen weeks through distance learning in a community where homelessness, child-headed households and absent parents are the norm seemed like an obvious impossibility.

Designing a workable distance-learning strategy with these contextual factors in mind was no easy task. Owing to low literacy levels of my learners and their parents, parents could not be heavily relied on for teaching purposes. Electronic learning would have been unfeasible due to the unavailability of electronic devices amongst learners and their parents, and in many cases, inaccessibility to the Internet and electricity.

I resolved to printing workbooks filled with lesson plans and worksheets for the 44 learners in my class, which had to be collected from the school on a weekly basis. However, communicating with my learners and their parents about collecting these resources, and the importance of doing so, presented yet another challenge. Although I prepared workbooks for every learner in my class for all nineteen weeks, on average, only two learners came to collect workbooks each week.

Being cognisant of the enormous ramifications that missing five months of schooling would have on my already academically-challenged learners, I was determined to have them be in possession of the resources. On many occasions, I drove into the heart of Epping Forest and The Range, which are two neighbourhoods which surround the school and which are riddled with relentless gangsters and soaring bullets, to deliver workbooks to my learners.

As a food-incentive school, approximately half of our learners rely on the Nutrition Programme as their primary source of food. While the school is closed, this government-funded feeding scheme does not operate, which has left many children without food in the past. In 2019, I started a holiday feeding programme at the school which feeds 300 to 400 learners per day, and this programme provided meals to our learners every weekday and public holiday for five consecutive months once the lockdown was implemented. I used this as an opportunity to distribute uncollected workbooks to learners who came to the school to collect meals. However, I was only able to reach a handful of learners in my class in this way.

Couple the stringent lockdown regulations with the Department of Basic Education's (DBE) ever-changing directives, accessing my learners' work for monitoring, and providing learning support engendered great challenges. As a result, I was not able to cover even a fraction of the curricular content from Term 2.

Months of planning and preparation preceded the return of my Grade 5 class. Familiarising myself with the new Annual Teaching Plans (ATPs/TAPs), Temporary Revised Education Plans (TREPs), Programmes of Assessment (PoAs), trimmed curricula, Covid protocols and the inconsistent directives from the DBE and WCED was overwhelming and exhausting.

Once my class finally returned to school, they returned in groups on alternate days due to physical distancing regulations. Once a week, both groups came to school in shifts (platooning) so that School-based Assessments (SBAs) could be written without compromising the integrity of the question papers. To avoid crowding at the entrance and exit points of the school, and for screening purposes, starting and dismissal times were staggered, thereby further reducing teaching time by almost two hours per day.

Extremely high rates of absenteeism (up to 50%), inconsistent school attendance and multiple drop-out cases further exacerbated my workload and reduced my ability to cover the curriculum content effectively. Owing to minimal parental involvement and support, sending consolidation and remediation worksheets home with my learners to complete on their 'off days', as an effort to get through more content, proved futile as the activities would almost always come back incomplete.

Unfortunately, systemic barriers within the education system have made it possible for learners to progress to higher grades without meeting the minimum requirements for their core subjects. As a result, the 14 Year-in-Phase (YIP) learners in my class, and a few others who have very low literacy levels, will likely progress to Grade 6 without being able to read basic sight words, and in one case, without being able to write their own name.

Notwithstanding all the challenges presented by the pandemic, the new teaching environment also brought about some benefits. Reduced class sizes made classroom management significantly easier and reduced the need for multilevel teaching, as the process of dividing the class into groups was guided by learners' individual cognitive levels. Additionally, a trimmed curriculum afforded me the opportunity to teach and consolidate individual concepts more thoroughly and lessened the immense pressure to mark lengthy assessments. Furthermore, the cancellation of co-curricular activities and some workshops afforded me the time to prepare more interactive lessons and provide additional support to learners after school. The pandemic also promoted personal hygiene and introduced positive routines such as eating healthily, coughing into a flexed elbow, and the regular washing of hands.

Although a commendable curriculum, CAPS can be unforgiving in that there is little flexibility and room for deviation. If concepts are not taught sequentially, learners will achieve little success. The reason for this is that they will miss the rudiments of the concepts if they are not taught chronologically. The DBE's decision to remove Term 2's content entirely, and parts of Terms 3 and 4, will have lasting effects on the learners' conceptual understanding and academic performance for years to come. In a few years from now, Covid will have been forgotten about, even though the effects thereof will perpetuate for every learner and student for the rest of their educational careers.

This pandemic has illuminated many shortcomings within the education sector, which is not necessarily a bad thing. This should be viewed as an opportunity to address the deep-seated disparities which have long borne consequences on crime, poverty and unemployment rates in South Africa. We simply cannot allow an entire generation to be the effect of Covid-19. Our country depends on an alternative.

G N Tibane
Thulisa Primary School (Gauteng)

Teaching during lockdown felt life-threatening, yet opportunities for growth were presented. Educators were requested to teach across all the grades. The workload was minimised as more educators came on board. Four educators were instructed to do rotational teaching to provide additional support. Assessments could not be completed on time due to learner absenteeism.

Online teaching was not possible as parents and educators did not have access to the Internet. Parent information was not updated in normal times to have meaningful communication between teachers and the home. As a school, we encouraged learners to watch the educational Channel 317 on DSTV, but we could not establish whether they actually attempted to view the broadcasts. The only other way to deliver the curriculum was through the DBE workbooks.

When the learners returned, we had to make a few adjustments. The school had to change the timetables to teach only 11 periods a day and for five days in three weeks. Educators prepared work to be done at home. Sadly, this was not done despite learners being at home for days on end due to the new rotational school attendance roster.

We have managed to teach only 40% of the prescribed Annual Teaching Plan. Learners in all grades will definitely have gaps in their knowledge going forward, which will impact their academic achievement for years to come. Intervention could be done to try and salvage the interruption of the academic year, but I am not very optimistic about it.

Teaching through this pandemic was challenging, to say the least. Three words linger with me when I think of this experience – tolerance, patience and consideration.

Anthea Maree Fortuin
Parkdene Primary School (Western Cape)

Teaching under lockdown: to some a fairy tale but to others the beginning of what seems like an endless nightmare. Teaching at a less privileged school has taught me many things, but the biggest lesson was realising how blessed I am, not only as a teacher but as a human being.

You are privileged enough to work at a school if you can work from the comfort of your own home, teach virtually, engage your students. However, in the community where I teach, education was not one of the top priorities during lockdown. People had more important things to worry about, like where their next meal would come from. People's livelihoods were at stake, and they simply did not have the time or energy to channel to worry about schoolwork.

Little teaching took place during the lockdown since most of our learners and parents have no form of proper communication with the school – let alone the equipment required for online learning. The only online teaching that took place was through activities sent over WhatsApp to about 20% of the parents. Even this was difficult, as parents complained that they do not have enough data to download the activities all the time. Unlike the privileged schools, we felt like we were stuck in a rut.

At my school, we had to go back to the basics and distribute packs of printed work, which parents or learners had to physically fetch from the school. In the beginning, it worked well, and learners were eager and enthusiastic about receiving work. However, as time passed, fewer and fewer learners collected the materials, and our plan of action was rendered ineffective.

When our learners returned, the lack of teaching and learning from home was immediately evident. It was like when we first met them way back in January. My anxiety levels rose during those first few days as learners had no sense of social distancing. My fear had to take the back seat, as helping our learners get back on track was the number one priority.

Our biggest challenge after learners returned was absenteeism. Learners simply came to school when they felt like it. Many used the excuse that someone at home was sick, and they had to isolate. There was also no way of regulating the truthfulness of this. We, as educators, had to repeat lessons sometimes up to four times. It became frustrating because, on the one hand, we wanted all the learners to get a fair chance at proper learning. On the other hand, we also had pressure from the district and government to cover the curriculum and conduct effective assessments.

Towards the end of the term, attendance improved to around 80-90% of enrolments. Learners also came to school 2-3 times a week, limiting our contact time even more. We were instructed by our subject advisors to cover the fundamentals for each subject, with assessment in mind. We did our best, adjusting our teaching methods accordingly. For example, in my grade, we did not have learners writing down notes as before. We printed and copied the notes beforehand to save that time. We also focused on explaining the content in class and showing practical examples where necessary; learners had to complete most of the activities at home.

It now became a shared responsibility between teachers and parents to ensure learners were busy at school as well as at home. Most subject advisors provided strong guidance and course content, and we simply had the job of preparing the lessons and teaching it to our learners. This support gave us extra teaching time and saved time otherwise spent on 'admin'. Many of our district officials even helped with the compilation of formal assessments, lessening our load immensely. It would be nice if this kind of support continued post lockdown.

I have a newfound respect not only for myself but for teaching as a profession. I am now more convinced that mine is a calling, not merely a job. Even so, we were ridiculed, embarrassed, and called lazy for simply fighting for the safety of our learners and their families. One thing is clear, teachers are frontline workers with or without a pandemic.

CHANTEL BOTHA
Andalusia Primary (Northern Cape)

Andalusia is in a rural town, Jan Kempdorp, in the Northern Cape. The Northern Cape Province is the poorest province in South Africa, and the rate of unemployment is very high. We have 432 learners in the school. About 193 (45%) of our learners are known to have learning difficulties. Further, we have 287 (66%) applications for school fee exemption for 2020, which is an indication of the socio-economic circumstances of our community. In this challenging context, I have been teaching Afrikaans Huistaal Graad 4 and English First Additional Language Grade 4.

Lockdown teaching was challenging. Not all of my learners had access to cell phones or the Internet, but as their teacher, I made a plan. I made hard copies and sent them to my learners. I communicated with 25 out of the total of 33 parents on WhatsApp. I send voice notes and exercises to the parents. I made use of my British Council resources, pre-recorded DBE Workbook stories. The learners loved this as they could hear the correct pronunciation. I also used YouTube videos to explain certain concepts. When the learners returned to school, it broke my heart to see how many were left behind since they did not have access to the Internet or money for data. I could see how many learners did not complete the work and I felt sad that the department had failed my learners; in my small group eight learners had no access to be able to work during the lockdown. Children suffer because there is poverty, joblessness, and there is very little money in these households.

I started a campaign called "Keep girls in school", where I liaised with businesses to sponsor sanitary wear for the girls in our school. I did this to curb the rate of absenteeism during the menstrual cycle of the girls. During the period that there was no school, I still made it available to our girls.

What saddens me the most is that some learners really have the potential but were left behind because their parents could not work during the lockdown. Learner X's mother is a single parent without financial assistance and could not buy data to be able to get work. The learner resides in the township far away from school and town. I went and dropped off hard copies at their shanty for her to be able to keep up with the rest of the class. Driving to her shanty, I became aware of the lack of services and opportunities in the township.

Learner Z has illiterate parents, so they are not able to assist their children with schoolwork. They live on a social grant and cannot make ends meet. It makes it very difficult for the learners to be supported if the guardian or parent cannot read and write. I started a homework period directly after school once the classes resumed to try and uplift these learners. It is tough in rural areas to teach where there is no support from the home. I also sell oranges and the money collected from that is used to assist learners in need.

Being a single parent myself, I am aware of the challenges of making ends meet. In my situation, during the lockdown, I went to school and made arrangements with the parents to come and collect departmental workbooks and hard copies of the work I had placed on social media. It is the only way I could try and get some work to my learners at home.

In my teaching career, I have started as a reading coach while I studied towards realising my dream of becoming an educator. I have empathy for these learners. I was awarded the third position at the National Teachers Awards in the category 'Excellence in Primary School Teaching'. I am also on the Provincial Task Team for Afrikaans Home Language. I was also invited by the British Council to write a short story for them. I am passionate about teaching and would like to be promoted where I can have a more significant impact on educational matters.

I wish that every learner be granted equal opportunities to achieve success in education. Lockdown once again proved that the elite was able to provide opportunities for their children where the poorest of the poor only fell further behind.

Nathan Stephens
Mitchells Plain Music Academy (Western Cape)

The eery part of 2020 was the persistent pandemonium of a scary pandemic. I started following the news of the novel coronavirus closely in late January. I saw the effects it was having on countries with established healthcare systems which left me very worried for my fellow South Africans and our beloved country. I immediately launched into research on online teaching methodologies that would help me be a little more prepared when the lockdown commenced.

Teaching music in schools and with organisations that facilitate music lessons through after-school programmes in under-resourced communities, I have had the opportunity to see the complete opposite ends of the spectrum. On the one hand, certain learners were privileged to have an instrument, an internet connection and access to a smartphone, tablet, or laptop. On the other hand, many other learners did not have an adequate combination of the above items at their disposal. Teaching music to children who had little to nothing was my greatest challenge.

After navigating some technical difficulties with online teaching platforms (which ultimately resulted in using two different apps simultaneously), I eventually found my rhythm. I enjoyed the benefits of literally having my classroom in the palm of my hand. When online teaching commenced, I reduced all my lesson times to 30 minutes per student, firstly as a data cost-saving initiative but mainly as a way of encouraging learners to manage their practice times efficiently. I have seen increased practice frequency from the majority of my learners as shorter practice sessions were encouraged. This was tracked on practise journals/logs, which were also converted to an online system, thanks to Google Classroom. Learners were able to post video clips or voice recordings from their practice sessions. Parents and peers were full of praise for these arrangements, with the result that my music learners had their confidence boosted. They were now more enthusiastic about music practice, and I was simply delighted as their teacher.

The external body, which moderates grading in Music, had to suspend the mid-year examinations due to the lockdown, but planned for an additional exam in early 2021. I have a few learners who enrolled for external theory exams, and we are looking forward to gaining exceptional passes.

The learning support offered by teachers working in the after-school space is often undervalued, but their contribution made will be extremely impactful in learner's lives for years to come. Every day, thousands of learners go home to no support or structure, but the offerings of After School Practitioners often assist in bridging academic gaps and offering social security from turbulent community environments. Many of these after-school interventions were suspended due to Covid with negative consequences for learners.

I have been a part of a fundraising initiative to assist in attaining resources for deserving learners who are not able to afford music lessons. We successfully hosted an online show during October involving a few of our learners and planned to host another online show which was live-streamed in December 2020.

More often than not, I tend to delay starting goals as the plans are not as perfect as I want them to be but teaching under lockdown has taught me not to wait until everything is perfect to begin working towards that goal, and I have basically summarised it into this one phrase: "Don't wait for great."

Kim Thompson
Bridgeville Primary School (Western Cape)

The lockdown announcement created quite an uproar with the abrupt closure of the schools. Fear and anxiety stalked parents with their children staying at home. This is quite tough on us as teachers because we could not 'wrap things up' and there was no proper 'send-off' for the holidays.

My school makes use of ClassDojo for communication. I have 31 learners in my class, of which only 16 parents were registered. Half the time when I posted notifications, only half of those 16 parents responded. When I noticed what was happening with absentee learners, I created a WhatsApp group with parents. This was the best way to stay in contact with my learners and I could send work through to them. At this point, I was not worried about using my personal number because the priority was getting through to the children.

It was not easy. I teach English, and my Grade 5s were the last learners to return to school after nearly six months of being home. I was insulted by parents for how I handled certain issues on the WhatsApp group and was even reported to the principal. I decided to "kill them with kindness", and things improved since then.

Luckily for me, I have a whiteboard mounted in my daughter's room, so it was ideal for teaching concepts and making videos using the board. I had brought all the required textbooks home and would take photographs of chapters or concepts and send it to the learners. I also spent a lot of money on mobile data because we do not have uncapped Wi-Fi. By the 10th day of the month, my data would be depleted because I used it to download YouTube videos and PDF documents that could assist learners to grasp concepts better.

It was difficult to manage all the changing requirements for teachers. It was expected of us to teach the Grade 7 learners when they returned and we had to assist my own class virtually. I complained about this because not only did we have to teach in the Grade 7 classes, but we also had to support our own classes, which I felt should have taken preference. I eventually told my parents that I would not be able to assist them daily and created time slots for questions and answers. We also created work packs for learners to work through, and this helped them because of the way it was structured.

When the Grade 5 learners returned, I was relieved because by then, I was tired of helping out and assisting in other grades. We worked on a booklet system where the work for the term as per departmental instructions was nicely structured. I found this very helpful because learners were able to cross-check the booklet's content with their DBE Blue Books and textbooks. When it came to the assessment, they were able to study from the booklet because we were told in virtual workshops that only work covered in the class could be assessed.

I am currently doing my B Ed Honours in Computer-Integrated Education. The transition from face-to-face instruction was therefore easy because I was already using online tools to enhance teaching and learning. The only difficult part was not knowing whether all learners were being reached. I eventually did a check-in where I would call the learners and find out how far they were with the lessons and whether they were coping. At this point, many parents were struggling financially or had become infected or affected by the virus. These difficult circumstances meant that little to no learning was taking place at home.

Some of my colleagues and my husband often say, "Jy doen te veel vir die kinders en hul ouers" (you are doing too much for the learners and their parents), but this is who I am, going beyond the call of duty and doing what I must to bring out the best in my learners (and people in general).

You develop a bond with the children. It was therefore difficult to monitor their progress or do a physical check to see if they were well or up to date with their work. I also missed out on their birthdays and other special events. I learnt that some of my learners were struggling to cope emotionally with their parents or family members being infected by Covid-19; some family even passed away because of the virus. With all this going on, some of the learners developed a sloppy attitude towards school because they were away for too long.

Others were resilient. I had one of my learners enter two competitions and despite his experiences of Covid-19. He won both, winning R300 and R350, always making waves for the school, the district and the province. This was an awesome achievement, but I was not able to celebrate it with him because his family was affected by the virus. He was moved to his grandmother's house for his safety. Unfortunately, his uncle then passed away too. It was very sad for him and all I could do was send messages.

I gave up my personal space when I moved to the WhatsApp group because parents were able to see my statuses and when I was online. This was a bit annoying, because often I found parents sending messages late at night and complaining about the fact that I was not responding to them. It also imposed on my family time because my phone would constantly go off, and even though I had teaching time and/or time set aside for questions and answers, parents still did not respect the times announced for communication.

I used PowerPoint presentations, PDF activities, and YouTube videos to extend the lessons. I did use the whiteboard. I also had bi-weekly Zoom meetings to explain lessons and check in with learners to find out how they were doing. For those who could not afford data for Zoom calls, I used WhatsApp video calls to see them.

For the Grade 5 learners, the lockdown situation was so overwhelming because they returned on 31 August with assessments starting on 28 September. This meant that there were only four weeks of teaching time which in effect amounted to only eight days. Then of the eight days, some of the learners would stay absent for one or two days. The fact that the year mark weighting was 80% made it possible for a learner to progress to the next grade even if he/she was struggling academically. Sadly, this is what we are going to be saddled up in and beyond 2021, given the gaps in their knowledge. Teachers will have to reteach concepts from the previous grades.

When Term 4 came, we had met as a phase to plan and plot coming assessments. School reopened on 2 November, and once again, we only had three weeks of teaching because assessments started in the last week of November. Our English department has set up oral assessments and asked learners to prepare from home because time was against us. We, also in accordance with Covid protocols, had to leave learners' assessments untouched for 24 hours before they could be marked.

At our school, we split the learners according to ability so that we had a strong group and the weak group. I found that with the weak group, you can do an intervention and get them on par with the strong group, but they are the ones that do not do homework and who give a lot of behavioural problems, so we end up spending a lot of time disciplining and, in the process, losing teaching time.

I already told my Head of Department, the type of child (academically) who will be coming to Grade 6 would be a direct reflection of Covid-19 and lockdown. She laughed and said she could say the same for the next grade because there are so many gaps. The Covid curriculum was re-designed to accommodate the learners, but learners were not playing their part.

In my class of 31, I had 20 learners who were not going to return. When the Grade 5 learners were due to return, I had five learners who stayed home due to comorbidities or the illness of a family member. The Grade 5 educator who was off on special leave availed himself to teach those learners who were learning from home virtually. This was great, for he did the same work that we were doing in class. In turn, we had to teach his learners.

With regards to attendance, every day I had a full class, reaching a maximum of 20 per class due to the halving of classes. We encourage our parents to screen the children before they come to school to avoid infections and to safeguard themselves and ourselves. Despite the absenteeism due to illness, most times, attendance was excellent.

Because of lockdown, I was able to build better relationships with learners and parents. It created a personal platform where things are shared on profiles or statuses and it gave me a unique opportunity to see what actually happens at home. It created a platform for my learners to be exposed to more than what they were used to in the classroom; they would also encounter a range of different teaching strategies. Most of all, I was able to get some of my learners to rise above their challenges and emerge more resilient from the lockdown experience.

Lehlohonolo Mofokeng
Saint Bernard's High School (Free State)

My body was taking strain from the often unreasonable expectations placed on us by district officials, with limited support. I knew that the announcement of the lockdown extension would spell trouble for my learners. I knew that the little momentum I was starting to build with my Accounting class was out of the window.

I wish I could say I was wrong. Akin to most sports, success in teaching hinges on the mutual understanding and trust between a teacher (coach) and learners (players). Since our physical proximity was compromised, I began to feel a deep sense of detachment from those I taught. After all, how do you begin to teach them from the heart when you have lost the emotional connection with them? How do you begin to speak to their hearts when theirs are detached from you?

As a township teacher, I relied on the school environment to provide the much-needed structure and routine for learners whose socio-economic realities often act as an impediment to academic achievement. Now I had to reinvent my pedagogic approach so that they would not lag behind their peers in the more functional schools. My efforts to bridge these learning gaps would face obstacles.

The reality where I teach is that children came from social and economic contexts where having food on the table ranked higher than buying data. I also had to make peace with the fact that even those who could afford data were not going always to be able to on a consistent basis. This realisation often left me feeling hollow and hopeless as a teacher. What made things worse was the sight of learners from opulent schools having their education uninterrupted because their parents could afford uncapped data bundles, or their schools had data funds to cater for the few who might have had difficulties accessing the Internet.

To make up for these inequalities, I started to record video and audio lessons which I would later distribute to my learners. As the saying goes, desperate times call for desperate measures. Because the lockdown regulations did not permit moving from one neighbourhood to another, I found myself sneaking around to meet with some of my learners' parents to share lessons stored on memory stick devices.

I also tried WhatsApp groups, and this intervention never really worked for the majority of my learners. Imagine sending three-page long notes on bank and creditors reconciliations to a group of learners whose English proficiency is not particularly high. Large proportions of my learners grasp the subject matter better through direct peer and teacher interaction in a live classroom. Stuck at home, they found it hard to understand the accounting topics I shared in our WhatsApp group. I would come to value the physical classroom structure even more.

Two months into the second academic term, the schools were closed again. A revised school calendar shifted education to the third term. This meant that I had to set aside whatever I had covered with my Grade 11 learners in the Term 2 curriculum. At the same time, there were calls from our district office for schools to administer outstanding formal tasks from Term 2, together with those planned Term 3. I do not see how this was humanly possible, for such workloads would surely come at huge costs to the health of teachers.

I remember how in the space of three days, I had to tell my class that the topic we were busy with the previous day was no longer part of the Annual Teaching Plan (ATP). I must admit, though, that this exposed the poor communication channels that already existed between the district, our school and us as colleagues in the commerce department.

Nonetheless, I am proud that I was well on track to cover the curriculum before my learners sat for their final exams and, like their peers in opulent schools were able to write a fully-fledged examination paper. Despite all the health risks, all the learners that I teach showed up for school throughout this stormy period. Equally miraculous is also the fact that these learners will not experience a significant gap in their academic knowledge of accounting in the next grade.

Young and talented teachers often choose to teach in well-resourced former white schools. This means our disadvantaged children in rural and township schools end up being starved of some of the brightest teaching minds, meaning they seldom get the opportunity to experience quality education. With the stark inequalities in mind, the lockdown period strengthened my resolve to one day build a world-class township school where children from poor economic backgrounds can access top-quality education that not only enriches them intellectually but also socially and financially.

4.6 Privilege

> "Tragically, the education system failed many schools in South Africa ... We were fortunate and enjoyed regular calls with heads in schools around the world where we shared experiences and learnt from one another."

FARZANAH EBRAHIM
Plumstead Preparatory School and St. Anne's RC Primary School (Western Province)

Dear Diary,

It is day 53, and we are still here. Still in our homes. Still being told to be good South Africans and still being told to live this life of 'social distancing'. What a terribly ironic twist life has taken. We are social beings by nature, but we are now being instructed not to socialise. Our entire lives we have been conditioned to make friends, to be cordial, to speak to our eccentric neighbours and to bond with our sometimes much to be desired relatives but now suddenly, we need to distance ourselves? Even more ironic is that once, I could not have enough of my phone and would look for every possible opportunity to scroll and type and Like. Now, every time I switch on a device, whether it be the TV, the radio or even just Facebook, I am bombarded with statistics, with pictures of people dying and with appeals for more funds.

While I sincerely do feel for all these suffering individuals, I also feel ever so alone and even more overwhelmed because no one ever talks about what it is like to be a middle-class schoolteacher stuck in a worldwide pandemic. But why should they? Why should they care about the white collars who are still so comfortable living in the suburbs with their Premium Netflix packages, pantries stocked with treats and, unlike the vast majority of South Africans, can still work from home? In the eyes of the world, there is no room for even an inkling of pity for us middle-class adults with our good health and steady teacher incomes. To the world, we are just getting a free pass to saunter about aimlessly in our cosy three-bedroom simplexes, where we can use a conference call in our PJs and as a bonus, the canteen (also known as *the kitchen*) is the best it has ever been. It is a *homecation* where you finally get to try out your culinary skills making banana bread or Dalgona coffee, binge-watch a TV series, and spend the rest of the time recuperating. At last, we do not need to contend with screaming children and government baseline assessments. So, to the world, we teachers are getting paid to do nothing. But is it really the *homecation* it claims to be?

No, it is not, and do you want to know why? Because being a middle-class citizen teacher during a world pandemic is like being the middle child. You are so neglected and are often left to fend for yourself. You are too poor to live opulently, so you still have to stick to a tight budget because you are in limbo with regards to your school and their finances; on the other hand, you are far too rich to get a grant. Your mental and emotional well-being is just being quietly shelved because, like every middle child, your parents assume that you will be fine, so you are forced to build this tough outer exterior. Your parents, or in this case the government, needs to concentrate on the donations of the rich. Like the privileged firstborns, they dote on them and the babies. They need to envelop them with their wings of protection.

But what no one knew was that when I, your typical middle-class teacher, woke up this morning, I was as uncertain about my future as the next person. Will I still have a job at the end of the month? Will this e-learning actually work? Is my salary also going to take a nosedive? Will my students have a learning gap for life? What about all the expenses and projects that I am committed to? No one will give me a grace period. The government will never give me R350 to pay for my insurance or, at the very least, data to continue educating the nation. Then a voice lingers at the back of my head, "Oh wow, no money for insurance, but did you think about the millions of South Africans starving today while standing in trailing lines just to get a basic piece of bread?"

I then throw that self-pitying thought away because that is what a good citizen will do, for I accept that I am better off than millions at the moment. After my moment down the rabbit hole, I realise that I need to start with my own child's online learning classes for the day because I am rich enough to afford data, but not rich enough to forfeit the school year. My kids need a career when all of this is over, so Corona or no Corona, they need to go back to school once schools reopen. To add to the pressure of the day, I also need to complete my own day of teaching because, again, being a middle-class citizen, I teach at a school that can afford the online teaching platform. To make things worse, the saddest irony is that these individuals who can actually still afford school fees are jumping on the Lockdown Gravy Train so have decided, "Well, I just will not pay school fees until we are back at school." So, a little bit more stress because if no fees are being paid, that means that there will be no salary for me, but here I am, still completing the syllabus so diligently every day.

Being middle class, we are not subsidised by the government, but I hear the government workers are not only getting paid their full salary each month but are not even expected to work or teach … so perhaps I am on the wrong side of the food chain. In any event, the entire morning goes by in a whirlwind of classes with a constant flow of interruptions: no one ever warned us or at least eased us into this new concept of 'working from home'. I am using my own data to educate the next generation of South Africans. Once again, no subsidy from the government.

It is difficult having to contend with my family life and still get the job done; otherwise, there is no pay at the end of the month. I then need to prepare meals and a million other snacks because although I need to work, apparently I am a mother and wife first. My roles have blurred to such an extent that I honestly do not know what I am doing most of the time, and this is grossly imposing on my mental health. But I am a middle-class teacher, so it cannot be that serious, right? Wrong, because realistically speaking, no one can play this many roles and do this many things in this small of a space.

My next concern then is, what about the house? I do not have the means to hire a live-in domestic, but my house is not that tiny either. So, with my two womb gremlins tearing apart the house, I am constantly packing and cleaning and cooking and feeding and teaching and trying my hardest to maintain my sanity amidst it all. And just when I feel like it is over, I know this overworked, throttling monotony of a day will only resume tomorrow. But this does not matter because I am a *privileged* middle-class teacher.

And what will tomorrow bring? Another voiceless day from our leaders? Again, not rich enough to be privy to the inside information of any of the government officials, but also not destitute enough to be unfazed by what is happening. As the numbers rise, I have another fleeting moment of desperation. This oh-so terrible roller-coaster of emotions is something I contend with daily. I constantly go from do not worry this cannot last forever to what am I going to do when I get that much-dreaded letter at the end of month letter telling me that my salary will be non-existent?

Yes, I know this all seems so trivial in the bigger scheme of things. Others suffer more than me. I should be so grateful that I have a home, security, and my family. But is it also wrong for me to say that I am tired? That I am tired of being overlooked by my country? That I am tired of the uncertainty? That I am tired of my government not giving me a break and cancelling some of my instalments? Why does my grief have to be minimised and compartmentalised just because I am a middle-class wife, mom and teacher? People always say it is easier to be born without something rather than for it to be snatched away from you later on in life.

At this moment in time, I could not agree more. My family and I do not know this life. We are used to getting up early in the mornings to start another day at school, we are used to scrambling about trying not to forget this lunch or that project, and we are used to being in contact with others. I am also used to dropping my kids off at school and not having to refresh myself daily with Grade 3 Math. I mean, who really cares about fractions during a lockdown? I do empathise with the less fortunate; I do. But I also want the world to know that while the sentiments of a middle-class teacher will never make the front pages of any newspaper, I think I speak on behalf of many when I say: "Dear South Africa, although we love you so much, we are also so exhausted right now and would just as much want our old school lives back. Your middle-class teachers."

Robyn Klaasen
Private School of Cape Town* (Western Cape)

You would be forgiven for thinking that being part of a prosperous, international school is smooth sailing. In fact, that is often what these elite schools want people to think. However, if 2020 has taught us anything, Covid cannot give two hoots about who you are, where you come from, or what resources you have. As a result, the effects of the pandemic on our school, although different from many other schools, has still been significant and disabling.

I am a high school teacher. I teach Health and Physical Education to all grades and a course called Independent Projects for Grades 11 and 12. I am also in charge of all non-academic campus activities. By all accounts, my department is not nearly the most important in secondary education, so I imagine that you could take my account and multiply it a few times to get a glimpse of the effects of the pandemic on the core subjects.

We started lockdown teaching with a two-day crash course on the online tools we would need. We were familiar with Google Classroom but had to add Zoom, ScreenCastify, PearDeck (to name a few) to our arsenal because the expectation was that we would conduct both synchronous (online, in live time, with our full classes) and asynchronous (offline, self-study) learning for our students. Can you imagine doing Physical Education like this? Thank God for phone cameras and people like Joe Wicks!

Anyway, what followed was a desperate search for online content, hours and hours of late-night prep – because I have three kids too, who were also all doing online school during the day (yes, in between my own classes) – and lots of weekend work. It is a funny dynamic: you gain time with things like not having to travel and being able to start dinner during break times, but you lose the distinction between work and home. When you spend every day in a 'presentable' top and pyjama bottom, the weeks eventually blend into a never-ending combination of both home and work without the benefits of or relief from either. Stress and burnout came nicely wrapped in adrenalin.

Here is another thing: just because you work at an 'affluent' school does not automatically mean that you yourself are an affluent individual. My Wi-Fi (which I acknowledge is a luxury not everyone has) was not suitable for online teaching, let alone simultaneous online learning (no one tells you that it is the upload speed you need to look at for live online communication). I regularly dropped calls and quickly realised the need for pre-recorded material. A surprising number of our students experienced much of the same. I may have disregarded some of my professional boundaries and used WhatsApp a couple of times.

While I am honest, I can confess that I took some liberties with the curriculum too. There is no way you can substitute the mass teaching, five-sensory feedback, and class interaction of in-person teaching with the online alternative. Between legitimate absenteeism, 'broken' cameras, and radio silence, you are lucky if you can complete 50% of the lesson. Not to mention the time required for students to submit work and the even longer time required to grade and give feedback on it all. Some subjects are lucky: you can leave out some of the detail and still meet the course objectives and standards. Others simply cannot. Our school adopted a practice of grace over grades, understanding the fragility of our students during this time – but even this had a sell-by date because at what point will this grade impact overall averages, thereby influencing a course of events that students and parents vehemently believe will be make-or-break them for the rest of their life?

I admit we were fortunate in many ways – and here is evidence of an unequal system. As a result of our northern hemisphere calendar, we did not experience much shut down because we are an independent school. Our kids could continue learning. However, we did ask questions about our own safety as teachers during these times, as we were expected to be on campus teaching (while our children in local schools were locked down at home). You would have thought that other community members may have had these concerns too. However, when our school was open, we had 70% in physical attendance, with most of those attending virtually; doing so as a result of being stuck outside of the borders or having comorbidities. And you would think that with those high numbers, you could almost continue with business as normal (minus the PPE, social distancing, constant cleaning of hands and space).

Enter Dual Delivery – the decision that each class taught live, on-site would be simultaneously broadcast for the students who could log in online and recorded for those students who either could not or were in a different time zone. For any practical subject, this basically means developing and running two parallel courses – one on campus and another virtually – because there is no way you can replicate a music class or science experiment in someone's living room. And do not get me started on the complication of someone returning to campus halfway through a term! It also means your work hours could extend around the clock because if you want face-to-face learning time with someone who could not make a class, you have to meet with them at another time. One of my colleagues taught Math from America, on Zoom, in the middle of the night (for her) – a major win for technology and education, though probably a loss for her mental well-being.

If you ask a teacher about teaching during or after lockdown and do not mention or allude to the fact that they were (perhaps still are) absolutely shattered, they are dishonest or delusional – send help! The physical, mental, social, and emotional impact is immense, and the sacrifices required not only by the teachers but also by their loved ones are immeasurable. But teachers would not be teachers if they did not find some silver lining in every situation. Here is just some of what lockdown taught me: Teaching is a calling. There is not enough money in the world to keep someone who is not inherently passionate about people and education in this business. I was not sure about this calling for myself, but I have seen my own eyes light up as the penny drops or a student takes the time to thank me for my efforts.

Education is not just important to parents and teachers. Students want to learn. Ours had the option of reverting to virtual learning at any time. None of them did. They even endured three hours of physical torture, I mean, physical training per week to do so. This year has shown just how persevering, determined, and resilient they can be.

We have, in our diversity, realised that we are actually the same. We all need a place where we are safe, loved and valued. We all experience hurt and loss. We all are holding on desperately to the hope that we will survive this. And when we have realised this, we would have been able to find love, friendship and support in the most unlikely places.

As I write this, we are on summer break, still approaching the peak of the second wave. To imagine that lockdown learning is a thing of the past would be foolish. We can only learn from what we have done before and adapt what we can do better. When you consider the rate at which things change, there is only so much that can be prepared in advance. We cannot assume that anyone really knows what to do or that we will not mess up royally before this thing is over. All we can do, is be kind – to our students, parents, colleagues, and ourselves. We are in this together, after all.

RENE FAHRENFORT
International School of Cape Town (Western Cape)

Thirty-three years of teaching provided me with the confidence to tackle 'all things teaching and learning'. After all, I am fearless, feisty and fabulous as a teacher, right? My teaching stripes were earned from Lansdowne to Factreton to Garlandale to London to Wynberg. Seriously. What could possibly unsettle this teacher?

When the lockdown was announced, my line manager provided training on how to prepare lessons and teach remotely. We attended training sessions on how to use pretty much everything available to teachers. There was provision made for children to collaborate on slides – each child in their own home and slides were to be differentiated; you name it, we were trained in it. We loaded our car boots with tripods, cameras, iPads, flipchart paper, markers, and some teaching equipment that we thought we might need down the line. Driving home, I was excited about 'all this time'. I would finally have to do a million things I never get to do in term time.

Initially, we 'just' uploaded work to Google Classroom – that was a marginally palatable daily task. We then needed to step it up a notch and include Zoom meetings with the children. This was where my 'vocab' started supersizing. "Zoom sessions" became synonymous with "send me the link", "sign in" and "join". Slideshows and other types of presentations then needed a more personal touch, and Loom was another thing I learnt about very quickly. It was all downhill from there as it was now about plug-ins, extensions and add-ons. The hamster was on the wheel and the brakes were failing. Cordless mouse in one hand and bruised teacher ego in the other, yet still trying to smile and wave.

The rate at which my vocabulary expanded is comparable only to the literal, personal growth that I experienced as a result of my successful attempts at walking in the light of YouTubed Fatima Sydow videos. Cooking now equated to meals laden with not so simple sugars. Lockdown was a Google education fest and a carb-fest. With the benefit of hindsight, my response to me not really knowing exactly what I was doing each minute of each teaching day was to cook and eat; there were days when it felt like I inhaled the food. If Springbok colours could be awarded for comfort eating, then I would certainly be sporting that green and gold blazer right now. The Siya Kolisi of comfort eating.

Back to my ever-expanding 'vocab'. So many verbs could be used as nouns and vice versa. This is huge in the world of a 'words person' like me. Hangouts, MS Meets, Zoom, Loom, Flip-Grid, add-on, plug-in, extension, submit via stylus, merge, convert from, convert to, split doc, hybrid teaching.

Enter the minor matter of being a single parent to a mildly-schoolwork-phobic teenage boy, who now *had* to sit in front of his laptop all day, while his mother was figuring out how to "sync", "attach", "upload", "send", "record" and "set", compounded the rabbit hole that was fast becoming my world. Who does that? A teenage boy, uncapped Wi-Fi, and a bedroom that became the classroom. A bathroom break meant passing the fridge; I could feel my eyebrows aching and going grey.

I soon realised that lockdown had become my teacher. I learnt that I needed to let go, allow it, go with the flow – all those peculiar things that other people usually did. Me? I planned, I envisaged an outcome, I went for it – with Plan A, B and C in my back pocket. In my world, there was progression, extension, monitoring and reflection. In that uncharacteristically quiet and deserted world outside my front door, there was a global pandemic, so none of my decades-old stash of learnt behaviour was really going to cut it. Interestingly, my teenage boy (who happens to be at the same school as the one I work at) thrived during this time of isolation. I did the best I could by the children that I taught. Mostly it was effective. They were some of the longest hours and the hardest work I have ever done, but it was effective.

I am now cheekily wondering whether the country was waiting on *me* to make a move to the types of teaching that our children need. I had not heard anything about how things will change, how teaching will evolve. I know that evolution is necessary; I have had a taste of the results of never-before-attempted types of teaching – both as a seasoned teacher and as a parent of a child that learns differently.

No story about teaching under lockdown would be complete without acknowledging the blessings that are parents of the children I teach and who were and still are supportive and understanding, and colleagues who share everything from recipes to URLs to video clips that were made to show the narrator of this piece how to use Loom. Covid has taught me that it takes a village to be a teacher. I have since realised that teaching is not what I do. It is who I am.

Penny Alston
Reddam House Umhlanga Preparatory School (KwaZulu-Natal)

We were excited about the start of the new school year. We had plans, after all; bonding, sports tours, the Moonlight Carnival, the School Production, the Grade 3 concert, Sunset Proms and much more. There were lots to look forward to, especially for our Grade 7s and their excitement to finish primary school for the last moments together. Suddenly the wind changed direction, and we reset our sails, forced by a storm into a context we did not imagine.

The students, staff and I felt like Alice in Wonderland teaching and learning in a new context. It was surreal, stepping back in time into a twilight zone, into a strange parallel world of school that we paradoxically knew well but did not at that moment. Like the students, we started those initial virtual lessons with mixed feelings of excitement and anticipation. They were fraught with anxiety, emotion and tears. Whatever lens we used to view the new normal, one thought remained constant in our minds: "When can we get back to school as we knew it?"

Our experiences challenged us, and we began to question ourselves, our values, what was important in life and who we were as individuals. We felt uncertainty in the new school environment. We clung to an in-built sense of order. This sense of order was soon put to the test by load shedding, internet connectivity and students using different devices for online lessons. Above all, the staff felt a real concern to maintain relationships with our students, whom we noticed grew quieter as the weeks continued. The silence of their voices was deafening. Fatigue also set in with increased screen time.

Just as Alice strives to create order from disorder, we had to transform unknown things into known things and locate strategies that would keep our students motivated. Chaos, by its very nature, is impossible to control completely. In those early heady days, as we entered into our own chaotic world, we collectively decided to avoid hankering after what we were used to, but instead use the pandemic as an opportunity to focus on authentic, active, compassionate and lifelong learning to help our students create an understanding of who they are. The first week of online connection with students left all of us feeling buoyed. "This is why we do our jobs!" we remembered. "It is not about the curriculum or the technology; it is about the students."

Our school has a reputable programme mix which is regularly subjected to robust accreditation, and a talented and dedicated staff who jealously guard our reputation as an independent school now also operating in virtual space. Tragically, the education system failed many schools in South Africa, and the chaos that was Covid revealed a complete absence of structure, a lack of clear information, and a cast of frantic characters. We were fortunate and enjoyed regular calls with heads in schools around the world, where we shared experiences and learnt from one another. In turn, we happily helped our public-school colleagues who phoned for advice on what to do, how to teach online and structure their new school day.

We have learnt to use many different tools to help us carry out the skills we can do easily in the classroom together. We have ventured into the world of Zoom, Seesaw, Microsoft Teams, Google Meets, Google Classroom, Google Docs, FlipGrid and Jamboard, and we will never look back.

School is about having fun and having fun in 2020 was more important than ever before. Our staff and students participated in the #JerusalemaDanceChallenge as a way to promote the message that we are stronger together. A pause in our school day for much-needed play and to show that together we can find ways to care, to learn, to hope, to inspire, to rise and to celebrate each other, to be thankful to be part of Reddam House, Umhlanga.

In a short space of time, a tiny virus turned the entire world upside down, leaving us to deal with the consequences for what will likely be a long time to come. As we navigate the remainder of 2020, it would serve us well to remember that grief wears many disguises, fear talks in unbecoming ways, anxiety gets controlling. At this moment, we are being called to love in ways we never have before. Our care calls to parents have confirmed these thoughts. It has been heartbreaking and humbling to hear their stories. All the staff and I can offer is the reassurance that we care deeply for the children, and our hearts are filled with compassion. The fourth term allowed for the resumption of traditional face-to-face interaction and a reorientation to reintroduce structure and rhythm into the lives of students and our school – and to make sure everyone felt safe and connected.

No one wished for this pandemic – and positive aspects only come with storm clouds. We have responded, constructively rethinking, in light of what we have learnt since March, about how school time might be better used. We are also buoyed by the enthusiasm of students both face-to-face and online, and we learnt a lot of new skills that will benefit our teaching in the long run, including how to have more fun. There are bright spots for us all in this brave new world. We are stronger, nimbler, more adaptable today than we were a few months ago. We have also come to understand what our children need more unstructured play, sunlight, nature, hugs, laughter, simplicity, daily rhythms and rituals, a clean environment, playtime with parents, compassion and expressed gratitude for who they are and believe in their goodness.

Mariëtte Wheeler
Protea Heights Academy (Western Cape)

Further in distance, even closer at heart – On the first day of lockdown level 5, a police van drove past the house, announcing: "You are under house arrest." I remember thinking: "No, that is not the correct terminology", but still a feeling of negativity, anxiety and uncertainty hung in the air. I realised that this would also influence my learners and knew that I had to be more sensitive to their emotional needs too, during this time.

I am a marine biologist who decided to go into teaching to share my passion for nature and, in particular, the marine environment with the new generations. As a new Natural Sciences and Life Sciences teacher, my focus was initially on teaching learners content. However, I soon learnt that more is achieved through building relationships with learners.

In 2020, I was teaching Natural Sciences and Life Sciences at Protea Heights Academy (PHA), a Maths and Science School in Brackenfell, Cape Town. I was also one of the nodal-school teachers for the new subject Marine Sciences that was piloted in 2020. At Protea Heights Academy, we were fortunate that we were already well equipped to teach online. From 2018, PHA was a Microsoft Certified School and educators continuously received staff development on various software. All learners were connected to Google Classroom for their respective subjects, with all our PowerPoint slides, videos, etc., being placed on this platform. We had a scheduled professional development session on a different topic planned for March. When the reality dawned on us that we would be teaching online, this training session was changed to exploring the various programs available to make online learning interactive and creative such as Padlet and FlipGrid.

My first lesson on Zoom seemed daunting, and I asked a friend and then my sister who lives abroad, to have Zoom sessions with me to familiarise myself with the program. After a few sessions, I felt more confident teaching in front of the laptop screen. Although most of my learners attended, I missed the connection with them as they were very quiet online. I realised that I had to bring more to the online classes and find ways to engage them to interact and ask questions.

While teaching, I always strive to make the concepts more than 'just textbook' to the learners. Where possible, I bring relevant material to the class or show video clips of real-life scenarios of the content. I therefore also carefully planned what I could use on the Zoom sessions. Fortunately, I was locked down at my mother's house in Lady Grey with a large, beautiful garden. For Grade 11 Life Sciences classes on flowering plants, I therefore had a variety of different flowers in front of the screen and could show them the various parts of the plants. For animal diversity, I even had a live earthworm in front of the screen to show them the different segments and movement of the worm. I even taught one of my Grade 8 Life Sciences classes while walking in the garden, pointing to various plants. In one of the online learning activities, I also encouraged learners to explore their own gardens, where possible.

Curiosity also increased attendance levels. In class, when teaching Grade 12s on the different forms of variation, my learners usually line up from shortest to tallest to demonstrate continuous variation. To still do this activity online, I requested on the class's WhatsApp group that each learner send me their height, along with various speculations by the learners of what I intended to do with this information. I received answers from 19 out of the 20 learners! I then searched for an animation drawing that made me think of each one of the learners and used these 20 images to create a line-up from the heights that they provided from shortest to tallest. Where I usually had 15 or 16 of my learners attending the online sessions, this session was even attended by learners who usually did not show up for the online class. The learners appreciated the image and understood the concepts that I explained. When we eventually returned to school, I made a colour printout of the image for each learner with a message of encouragement. I smiled when the final NSC exam paper contained a question on variation in learners' height.

One of my highlights that showed the need for learners to connect with me and their fellow learners also emotionally occurred in April. A girl in my Marine Sciences class had her 16th birthday. Her mother emailed me to ask if I could please do something special on the occasion. I therefore arranged a surprise for her by arranging with all of her classmates to have their videos on and have a card, balloon or flowers with them. The learners enthusiastically participated. With the Zoom Waiting Room option, I allowed everybody else in and then when we all "stood ready", let her in. She was overwhelmed by the special moment.

The first international World Albatross Day was hosted on the 19th of June. Before lockdown, one of the organisers and I planned to get my Marine Sciences learners involved in the event. Unfortunately, we could not proceed with the plans, but I still wanted to create awareness about these seabirds and their urgent need for conservation. The Agreement on the Conservation of Albatrosses and Petrels (ACAP) hosted the Great Albicake Bake Off and colouring-in competitions. Inspired by these competitions, I organised a Creative Class Competition for my Marine Sciences classes. Learners were tasked with drawing, painting, baking or making something creative "as long as there was at least one albatross included". Learners used what they had available at home and submitted images and photographs of their creativity online. The entries were scored online by independent judges, while learners were also asked to vote for their favourite. Poster and book prizes were sponsored by ACAP and the Antarctic Legacy of South Africa. Learners learnt about a real-life, current issue while using their creative talents – skills that are not always utilised in a scientific context.

On average, 70% of the learners in my senior Life Sciences and Marine Sciences classes returned to school on the allocated dates, while the majority of learners in my Grade 8 classes returned. While teaching in class, all lessons were still streamed as well as recorded. Video recordings were made available on a shared Google Drive afterwards. This allowed all learners the option to revisit lessons while studying for tests.

When learners were able to return to school, I was still very aware that the current situation affected them emotionally. In two of my classes, I placed Sticky Tags on the desks prior to class. I asked learners to write at least three words on the Sticky Tag on how they were feeling that day in general. I ensured them that I was going to be the only person to see the tags. From the responses, it was clear that learners were anxious, scared and uncertain. I informally followed up with each learner about his/her response. This gave the learners a channel to share some of their own concerns and situations with me.

As PHA teachers were teaching online throughout lockdown and getting learners to do various activities online, we managed to cover the entire curriculum in all grades for the Life Sciences components of Natural Sciences and Life Sciences. Most of the topics for Marine Sciences were covered in class, while arrangements were made with all nodal schools to have combined online classes in January to cover the topics that were trimmed. Despite all the online teaching, learners' performance at the end of the year was lower compared to previous years. This might have been as by departmental regulations we had to set tests instead of the formal exams in November. Also, in my opinion, this illustrates that for most learners, online teaching cannot replace a teacher in class.

On the last day of school for the Grade 12s, I felt very emotional. I realised that even more than other years, I walked a path with the learners. We worked together and struggled together through difficult times. I built strong bonds with learners in my other classes and will continue building these relationships in time to come. While it was important for me to teach concepts and terminology, it was just as important to me to get to know my learners and to give them the opportunities to use their creative talents. While lockdown forced us to be in our houses and at times it might have felt like "house arrest", it was a time when we grew closer at heart.

CELRI OLLEY
Mitchell House School Polokwane (Limpopo)

We have not only entered a time when we need to seriously reconsider the way in which we teach, but we have also been flung into a world pandemic where education itself is being politicised, and the fate of students and teachers lies in the hands of politicians and unions fighting for power.

Our mission has not changed, but how we approach what we do has. We have to change how we help students to reach their academic goals and ensure that we remain true to our own unique brand as teachers. We have to maintain our values and unique identity amidst the pushing and pulling of politics, policy, parents and fear. Now, more than ever, we need to stop and take stock of what and whom we need to be and become to ensure our students will never be referred to as a 'lost generation'.

My teaching journey started in 1999, but I found my teaching voice in 2014. Since then, I have devised my own professional development programmes to ensure I could keep up with sustainable trends in education, and that I could not only support my students, but also my colleagues on this journey.

Diving into the new normal believing that you have to master each new technology fad, attend every webinar course and take every online course that mentions remote learning and remote teaching is not only unrealistic, but it is the quickest way to burnout and loss of confidence in your own abilities and experience. However, to me, the 'next normal' is actually just another normal. The world is filled with change. Some changes are small and take thousands of years, while others are global and immediate.

I taught an extended 11-week term (which should have included a mid-year exam) without a single test. I usually teach inquiry-based lessons and I adapted these into 'chunked' one-week activities with specific feedback and daily connect routines that encouraged my students to engage. I was able to revise Term 1 work, to get them used to online learning, and then gently moved them into new work (their Shakespearean explorations). This meant I had to adapt the original plan substantially but keep the core skills intact. It was also the conclusion of our larger novel study and this also had to be re-thought.

I found that parents suddenly thought their older children needed to share their devices and become co-teachers and babysitters while they worked from home. I discovered that children not surrounded by other children learning the same things are more susceptible to distraction, and most importantly, I learnt that no executive access is possible when you work with children suffering from anxiety and stress-related withdrawal.

Some students were trapped in homes with alcoholics with no access to alcohol. Some were trapped in homes with abusive parents; others were trapped in homes with less access to basics such as water and sanitation or a warm plate of food. How could I expect them to stick to due dates if they had to walk three kilometres to the nearest cell tower to get mobile connectivity and then had to choose between which subject's work to download?

I work at what is described as a 'privileged' private school, and these were the very realities we were faced with as teachers and students. We (teachers) had to work around these and make plans, and approach management with issues, which they found amazing solutions for. Planning became a holistic, living activity that changed as the weather did, and we had to ensure we kept abreast of everything. The result was an even larger admin load, but we thought we had it under control.

In my circles, a lot has been said about assessment. Now is the time to move away from test-based assessments and into other options that require thinking, problem-solving, creativity. Tests now in this already stressful and uncertain time is like playing with matches in a flint factory. Just do not do it. You won't feel up to marking and they will not be able to study.

In the third term, we had some face-to-face time again, we had the 20/20 vision of hindsight, and we trimmed our admin and revisited how we approached certain situations.

Choosing what is important and what is not becomes the triage of the classroom. In this pandemic, I became the Next-Normal Teacher teaching through lockdowns. It is how we decide to deal with change that shapes how we grow into these 'next normal' paradigms. I remember the saying, "double the work in half the time".

4.7 Perspective (novice teachers, older teachers)

> "As a newly qualified teacher in a pandemic, I learnt that I have to be extremely flexible."

> "I found myself cut off from a teaching style I had been accustomed to all my life ... How was I going to do this?"

KIRSTEN COURTNEY DANIELS
SH High School* (Western Cape)

After my final year at varsity, I struggled to find employment as an educator. I was however fortunate to fill in at the school where I conducted my teaching practice. That school is one of the most well-run institutions I had experienced in my short life. If I could turn back the clock and the school existed, I am confident that if I were enrolled in this school as a child, I would have excelled academically.

I was hoping my teaching practice school would inform me when more permanent posts became available. After all, I showed up as a fill-in teacher at any time they asked me to. Sometimes, I would receive a message or call at 05:00 in the morning, asking me to fill in, and I would be there earlier than I should. I thought they would see me as one of their reliable and competent teachers, but I was mistaken.

After a while, the calls and messages became less. I was officially unemployed. I worked on my CV tirelessly, trying to make it as 'attention-grabbing' as possible and calling around every day but without success. I became despondent. Then, when lockdown happened, I gave up. I resigned myself to the fact that it was no longer possible to find employment and that nobody would employ me.

Miraculously, one Monday morning, I received a phone call from a school about 20 minutes away from me, asking me whether I was interested in starting the upcoming Friday. It was made clear that my contract would end in December. I was anxious but excited as well. I knew that I had to prove myself and that I would have to work very hard as I was employed in the middle of the second term, and the teacher had decided that it was time for her to retire. I could not be more thankful for her decision.

I remember I had to start on a Friday. I was told my duties were to teach Grade 10 English Home Language, Grade 9 Home Language, Grade 9 First Additional Language and Grade 9 Life Orientation. I felt excited and overwhelmed simultaneously. Then I realised I had no students. Not one. The learners would only be back a month and a week later. I started preparing their assessments, analysing their work to find out where they lacked and made notes for them so that they could read it before coming to school so that I could spend less time teaching that content.

I had to prepare but I had no idea what the learners were like, I had no idea what level they were on (academically) and, with a weak immune system, my anxiety started getting the better of me. I had sleepless nights just thinking about possibly contracting the virus from a learner. Screening learners and teaching with a mask were difficult. The school I am teaching at decided to phase in grades on different days in adherence to the lockdown rules. This resulted in seeing my learners once a week; with such limited time to teach and assess, it just felt impossible.

At the end of every day, I was exhausted. All I wanted to do was lay my head down and sleep. Then, I realised that I had to stand in the cold during the early hours of the morning to screen and sanitise learners. This was coupled with shouting over a mask whilst I was sweating profusely because I could hardly breathe in this mouth cover. The routine continued after school again. However, this time sanitising the desks at the end of the day formed part of our duties as we only have two caretakers. It would be unreasonable to expect them to sanitise every classroom we have used.

Once all the sanitising duties were performed, it was time to tackle the curriculum. Trying to fit half of the curriculum into a limited time schedule was challenging. I found difficulty having to teach the learners how to write an essay and then having them complete it in an hour. Not only did I have to cover the revised curriculum, but we were expected to teach them additional work to prepare them for the next grade, as my supervisor had instructed me. I decided to draw up a little booklet with everything they will be assessed on, especially the activities that were not included in the revised curriculum.

At this time, it came to my attention that my learners' levels of reading and writing were not close to what it should be. I decided to do "shared editing" to assist them with this skill because clearly, it was not something they were used to. The goal was to nurture writing skills and also help them read with comprehension, but the time was just too limited.

I found so much difficulty preparing lessons and assessments because our subject advisors would regularly send out new and changing information. As a result, I would have to reassess learners, and this set me back in my planning. What made matters even more challenging was the fact that most of our learners are from disadvantaged backgrounds and therefore teaching online was not an option. We would communicate via WhatsApp groups. Still, it was of little use as learners would either exit groups, not bother to complete the activities, or simply claim that they did not have data to download the files. It became frustrating and left one feeling despondent.

Not much teaching took place during this time as we had very little time and were expected to correct the previous term's work as it counted quite a bit towards their third term marks. Personally, it was frustrating since much of the assessments I had to cover with learners had to be done under controlled conditions. I could not allow them to do it in one part of the classroom with their peers, as I would have to teach in another part of the room and could not keep an eye on them. Sometimes the learners I was teaching would become rowdy, resulting in the learners doing the assessment becoming distracted. Nor could I do teaching and assessment work later in the day. The area I am teaching does not allow me to have classes after school as it is not safe for learners to work too late.

The school year really affected learners badly. Shortly after they returned, new lockdown regulations were put in place. Many students lost the motivation to come back and some of them developed the mindset that 'the teachers must make us pass'.

As a newly qualified teacher during this pandemic, I have learnt that I have to be extremely flexible and take advantage of every minute available with my learners. My mental and physical health were at levels I had never experienced before. Within the space of two days, I went from a middle-ear infection to bronchitis which set me back with my learners' progress with the result that I experienced panic attacks and sleepless nights. It honestly puts me in a panic seeing how far behind our learners are and how they are going to struggle in the real world academically.

University training did not prepare me for what teaching in pandemic times is actually like.

BENITA SOLOMONS
Yellowwood Primary School (Western Cape)

I resigned from my beloved profession in 1995. After being out of teaching for about ten years, I decided to reapply for a teaching post in 2007. Although I was pleased to be teaching at an early childhood development centre in the private sector, there was no job security.

I knew that it was not going to be easy, but how hard could it be? I am passionate about teaching and I love children. However, nothing could have prepared me for the change that greeted me on my return to the classroom. I had never felt so incompetent in all of my adult life. At home, my family would find me surrounded by files until the early hours of the morning trying to make sense of the new curriculum. If having to adapt to the new curriculum was not stressful enough, there was also this strange new technology to deal with. Gone were the days of writing by hand. I had to get used to words like a soft copy, hard copy, paper trail, etc.

I missed the days with the little ones where there was minimum planning and maximum playing. Learning through play was a thing of the past. The one thing that kept me going was the fact that I knew how to teach and that I loved my job. And that is precisely why I was still around in the classroom in 2020.

Then came Covid-19, and with it a threat to my health, my sanity, and my job. I had a lung disease at the age of 35, combined with hypertension, which almost cost me my life. Fearing this new illness, I applied for special leave. I doubted that it would be granted but was thankful when my application was successful. On the one hand, I was relieved, while on the other hand, I was petrified. This new way of life brought new challenges. Off-site, on duty, was my new stressor.

I am old school, so the blackboard and different colour chalk is my forte. When I was required to teach from home, I found myself cut off from a teaching style I had been accustomed to all my life. I was forced to move out of my comfort zone. I had sleepless nights. How was I going to do this?

Then a colleague of mine suggested Screencast O'Matic, which not only rescued my sanity but saved my career. I was back in business. I pre-recorded my lessons and sent them to the onsite teachers who were now required to teach our classes. Some of them had never set foot in a Grade 7 classroom. I felt bad for my colleagues, especially our HOD, because I could tell that all this pressure took a toll on them. Our head was the only Grade 7 educator at the school. The other two educators and I were granted leave to teach from home due to comorbidities.

My HOD and colleagues also suggested Zoom, but I decided to stick with what I was comfortable with. I could not bear the stress of feeling out of control and incompetent in front of my learners and colleagues. They would have been able to pick up my negative vibes. I slowly got into the swing of things, even enjoying some of the lessons, but it was never easy. At times I felt like returning to school, but the fear of contracting the virus kept me home.

It must have been very difficult for our learners, this new normal. They left at the end of the first term, only barely getting to know their new educators, only to come back to new teachers with only a quarter of their friends in the class.

The teachers were very concerned during the first few weeks because the learners were, as they called it, mute. I was glad when I heard that after seeing my recordings, they seemed to come out of their shell a bit. This brought tears to my eyes. I felt that I had abandoned them and prayed that the separation would be over soon.

On a more personal note, I realise now that I probably should have reached out to my colleagues more and not waited for them to make contact. I guess I was a bit scared of being criticised, given my own insecurities. Nothing beats physical presence, as what is being said on chats or messages can sometimes be misinterpreted. I really and truly appreciate the extra mile that my colleagues went for me personally. I could come back knowing that my learners were on par with other Grade 7 learners, although I was never there for them physically.

I was often paranoid that I was not doing enough from home and was very aware of what was said on our phase's group chat. I felt that I had to run through the day with them. I was scared of running out of data and not being able to connect with colleagues or school if they needed me. I never left my home during school hours for fear of being seen as not on duty. I would carry my phone from room to room in my house to be able to hear it go off if I was needed. Most of the time, I was not needed, but it was my own paranoia.

During the initial lockdown, when all educators were home, teaching from home was not that bad. The WhatsApp group with parents and learners seemed to work perfectly, although a few learners exited the group so as not to receive work. I do not know how much the teaching from home during the initial lockdown benefited our learners. The teachers were required to reteach the work on their return which I thought was a waste of valuable time which we could not afford. For those who were not able to access the work or the lazy ones who never tried, this must have been ideal.

It would be nearly impossible to recover what the learners had lost with the staggered approach we were following. Taking into account absenteeism, personal problems, and illness, to mention but a few, catching up seemed unrealistic at best. The learners who worked with the teachers during lockdown at least had a bit of an advantage.

Around 80% of Grade 7 learners returned to school in the first week after school reopened while the others returned gradually. The two-day, three-day cycle was problematic. Once a learner has missed his or her turn for the week, you lose them for the entire week, and there is no way for them to catch up on work.

The positive things that I experienced during lockdown were that I was forced to equip myself with the knowledge to be able to do most of my work on a computer. I had more time to study for the last lap of my degree, and I could try my hand at poetry. As far as us being on holiday, which was the general conversation amongst the public, I would have preferred to rather be in school and on duty.

KEMBLE ELLIOTT
Redhill School (Gauteng)

Lockdown surprised me. I mean, it took me by surprise, and I was surprised by my reaction to it. Like the first flattened and bent minor chord of the sax in a bluesy tune, it filled me with melancholic ennui. Anxious "What-if?"s and "How-long?"s butted heads with "It will be okay" and "I support the government's efforts. Thank goodness for CR."

"My fellow South Africans …" sounded like a fatherly blessing. However, the anxiety was visible in every gaze I met, whether it was the students in my well-resourced private school classroom, the teachers in the staffroom, or the hapless individuals standing at traffic lights with signs. I suddenly became aware of two things: that, no matter how different our means and opportunities, this pandemic situation was going to challenge us on a whole new level, and that those without would be far more challenged than I. I found myself bolstering my own insecurities and worries by showering others with inane platitudes: "It's going to be fine." (How did I know?) "It is what it is." (What a useless and meaningless phrase!) "Hang in there, you've got this!" (Like hell.) I also thought (hoped?) that lockdown would be three weeks at best. We could do three weeks, right?

We ended our first term of 2020 in the aftermath of the President's announcement, knowing that our holiday would be overwhelmed with re-planning (all right, starting from scratch) to accommodate different timetables, different lesson lengths, different groups of children, different means of delivery. Basically, we were expecting ourselves to keep everything the same, with nothing being the same in any way – an illusion of smoke and mirrors, as tenuous as the promises made in a dimly lit bar. We wanted to provide consistency and security for our students (many of whom were dealing with the spectre of Covid-19 in their homes and extended families) without in any way being able to keep things the same. I packed up what I thought I needed from my office and set up a new office space in the spare room of my home. My husband, who is also a teacher in a government school (which had its own set of problems that had to be managed), used another room, and our animator daughter set up her work computer in her bedroom. We were less than six metres away from each other at any given time, and yet we barely saw each other. This was a lockdown round one.

My matric AP English students happily used the WhatsApp group we had already formed, so we set up sessions and conversations that way. My matric IB2 Theory of Knowledge students were primed and ready to go, with extra twilight sessions that helped them complete the homework research. They responded best to the strictures of home learning, becoming more focused and better at time management. When Cyril called for lockdown, I postponed a project with my Grade 10 Life Orientation students (an oral which was due the following week). I reassured them that we would resurrect it once we were back at school – famous last words.

A week into the first term of lockdown online school (after three weeks of Easter holiday that did not feel like Easter and was nothing like a holiday), I sat at my desk, staring out into the verdant garden (aware of my privilege, again), wondering what it all meant. I was supposed to be working, but instead, I wrote a sonnet. The musings of a scattered mind:

> LOCKDOWN SONNET (1 week in)
> How quarantine will change the way we live
> Imagination cannot fully see.

We might the imposition quick forgive
Or strictures fight and wrestle restlessly.
The housebound thoughts our freedoms could dethrone,
Thus, quick enchaining cabin fevered needs.
Those selfish, petty, self-involved moans
A lens revealing malaligned weeds.
But, if our fears we take the time to still;
Unhitched from modern life, we gently turn,
Embracing sweet simplicities until
Antiquity's deep truths from soils we churn:
Original, bright insights, vistas new
Through freshly opened eyes, we will clearly view.

I so hoped that the world, and I, would learn something from this pandemic. There had to be a point, did there not?

I, the forever-networker, the outward-bound-is-better-than-homebound explorer, the restless, easily bored partner in our family, was flummoxed by the sense of calm and stillness I felt. I loved being at home. I loved working out in our garage, even though it got freezing on midwinter mornings. I loved being able to teach in pyjamas, as long as I brushed my hair and put on a little make-up. But I hated not seeing all my students' faces. I hated the lack of control for the students I was worried about ... those young people who struggle on their own. I hated not being able to read a million micro-expressions – the currency of cooperative teaching and learning used by any facilitator. The dreaded computer-screen-of-letters remained unfazed by my pleading to switch on cameras.

I found myself greeting students at the beginning of the lesson, checking that they had signed into the assignment on the Google Classroom (how grateful I was that we had been using it already), and then waiting around for questions, as the students worked alone or in small groups (sometimes in another online classroom, sometimes on WhatsApp groups). They often mediated each other's learning without much need for me at all. Sometimes a lone voice would emerge from the multicoloured letter-littered screen. "Ma'am, what should we do next?" or "Ma'am, are we on the right track?" and I would attempt to solve the challenge and set them loose to explore the rich topics of Human Rights or Existentialism or Epistemology again. How strange to teach without classroom conversation and banter? I realised that the majority of my teacherly skill had been poured into the preparation of online resources that they were now using, so independently. Was that it? The call and response of the blues song had found its way into my carefully angled (to avoid piles of paperwork) and well lit (to avoid highlighting the wrinkles on my screen-framed face) computer camera. Was it that easy to force change in education? Really?

Just as things settled into a rhythmic routine, the requisite chord progressions of the Lockdown Blues forced us into the second and third iterations of online school. Another timetable, split classes, repeated days, Saturday sessions for 'full-time online' learners, shorter sessions, and repeated revision to planning, deadlines and timelines ramped up the anxiety and exhaustion.

And then, Uncle Cyril's extended lockdown ... again. His well-intentioned greeting to his fellow South Africans started to sound hollow. An out of tune instrumental soloist. But we were allowed back to school. Almost. Half the students online, half in the classroom ... a new level of torture emerged. When you hear teachers say, "Never have we worked so hard"; don't for one minute believe that they normally have time on their hands. We do productions and magazines, galas, and social events, without blinking an eye in 'normal' school time (whatever on earth 'normal' is). Whoever said that teaching was a half-day job was completely oblivious to what teachers actually do, including nights and weekends of marking and prepping at home. But this, this was pouring every single iota of energy into 'being the best online teacher'. Doing it better ... going further ... being more available ... blurring the lines: between home and school, night and day, on duty and off. Jazzily improvising to cater for third and fourth timetables, we responded to extended lockdown orders, partial school return, hectic mask and sanitation regulations. All of which added to the stress and anxiety that everyone felt.

And let's not forget the added stresses of managing locked-down parents, who were stressed at having to manage locked-down students, who were stressed with not seeing their friends or having any of the usual markers of a school year (productions, sports days, matric dance), without being able to manage our own locked-down stress. An oft-repeated chorus in three voices, "Don't nobody understand my pain? Doesn't anybody ever understand my pain? Ain't nobody gonna hear me go insane?"

After 33 years in education, I was saddened by this last term. It was so challenging. So damned hard. My students and I managed to get tasks done and stay on course with the curriculum (and, let's be honest, the marks that show the world that we have done our jobs). Even the presentations that were suspended at the beginning of lockdown were squeezed in before the August holidays. The students bravely did things online, challenging themselves to work collaboratively and to meet deadlines (most of them ... most of the time ... mostly). All the marking was eventually done (in the holiday, of course) but still, we all survived (a thoughtfully chosen keyword). And the third term loomed.

I found myself thinking about the Persephone goddess of the underworld. A lot. That trip into the underworld, or more accurately that abduction perpetrated by Hades, was meant to symbolise the earth's withdrawal of sustenance as winter encroaches, allowing for inward-looking self-reflection until new growth bursts forth when spring returns.

How strange that we went into lockdown at the end of autumn and emerged as spring returned. Something mythologically significant has happened. Will the world, and I, use the lessons?

And it was at this point that I was fortunate enough to be offered the opportunity to leave teaching, to focus on the budding consultancy I (and two friends) had started. The second term of 2020 was my last term of teaching in a school. It was by far the most difficult of my career. More difficult than the first (in 1987), which has always stood out as an intense and wonderful baptism of fire. I am so grateful that I had this last term, though. It reminded me that teachers and students (and even parents) are the ultimate jazz musicians. The ultimate ensemble players, trying to bring together different perspectives and skills to produce something that emerges from the subterranean depths of pain and fear to reveal something beautiful, strong, and evocative. We played the Lockdown Blues.

TASNIM MURADMIA
IR Griffith Primary School (Gauteng)

Then came the pandemic. Teaching and learning as I knew it came to an abrupt halt. Everything changed. Being an educator for the past 22 years, I secretly rejoiced in getting an 'extended holiday'. That joy was short-lived as I realised what that meant in terms of education.

Education had to be reimagined, reinvented, and reorganised on terms set by the pandemic, and that scared me because I did not know where to start. I had to learn how to readjust the norms and standards of what a teacher did in the classroom to what a teacher had to do on a digital teaching platform. That is when I learnt that MS Teams was an acronym for Microsoft and not the non-existed word "Emes". Digital teaching was clearly not my forte.

My knowledge of technology in the classroom extends only as far as using a projector to teach a concept in a lesson in English or Maths by showing a video. Logging in, inviting groups of eight and nine-year-old learners was no easy task, especially since it took more time teaching them digital etiquette or how to mute and unmute their microphones than delivering the actual Maths or English lesson itself.

Thank goodness for patience, from both sides! I had to readjust my digital strategy and figured it was better to do my lessons on PowerPoint, then save it onto One Drive, convert the PowerPoint to a video and then save the video as a shareable link on the D6 Communicator for learners and parents to download and watch at their convenience.

The fact that I can write what I did is testament to how much I have learnt about digital teaching in Covid times, something I might never have done otherwise.

Honestly, the digital teacher never appealed to me or my learners. I realised that the need and comfort of having a human body in front of my learners outweighed the buffering and pixelated version of me on a screen. My kids simply needed to see me in real time, so I resorted to calling them individually on their parent's WhatsApp lines to talk to them. This was wonderful, and I instantly knew that the human touch of seeing their teacher was what my learners craved, far more than the curriculum.

Then came the curriculum. I was overjoyed at teaching a revised curriculum, something I had been advocating for years; there was so much unnecessary content in the pre-Covid CAPS curriculum. I could now focus on what my eight and nine-year-old learners needed; reading, writing, counting, and spelling skills which are the fundamentals of foundation phase education. Completing the curriculum was now less important than salvaging whatever time was left in the year for meaningful education in my classroom.

I was teaching from the heart to a class of 14 learners every alternate week. The children showed up diligently with brave faces, trusting me to teach and bring back some form of normalcy to their forever changed lives. I could see their fear of being in the classroom slowly fade away to be replaced with that hunger to learn and the desire to be a normal child in abnormal times. It remains scary and unchartered territory in education for everyone, but I saw it as a challenge worth taking on.

In the dreariness of a Covid classroom, I saw what an ideal classroom of 14 learners would be like, as compared to 40. I saw a glimpse of a class that was not overcrowded, where I could teach to every child's strengths and not just to cover the set curriculum.

Then came the parents. Parents now saw me, the educator, in a totally different light; there was definitely more respect. Before the Covid lockdown, parents were heard to say: "My child can do it with me at home, so I don't know why he can't do it in class." Now they say: "Thank you! I know what you mean now when you said my child is having difficulty." Validation, finally!

There was suddenly a rebirth of education, a reawakening of what it meant to be a teacher, and a realisation, sadly, of what we lost with our learners. No more hugs, or high-fives, no more let's play a game together, no more group work, no more watching kids just playing and being carefree on the playground. Each learner was now confined to a desk, with a mask or visor, staying put in little more than a one-metre squared block.

I had never worked harder in any of my years of teaching than in six months of 2020. Apart from my own fears of Covid and education, my mind was in a constant loop about what comes next. I cannot switch off, constantly re-evaluating and restructuring the small world of my classroom. I took comfort in knowing that I was doing my best for the learners in my class as they prepared to move to Grade 4 in 2021. There was a steady affirmation of our good work coming from my learners, parents, principal, and colleagues. I have become a better teacher. That is all I can do: to give my best and hope that it is enough.

SHAUNDRÉ-LEE BROWN
Yellowwood Primary School (Western Cape)

Nervous, scared and extremely anxious. These are but a few of the words that come to mind when I think back to the start of the lockdown. "What would happen to school, how would we go about teaching?" and, most importantly, "What would become of my learners? Will I ever get to hug them again?" As a new educator, it was difficult to wrap my head around everything that was going on, especially considering that everything came at us all at once. It honestly took me weeks to stop the chaos in the little personal box inside my head before I could even deal with my teacher box.

Once I got my mind right, innovation took over and I found myself working harder than ever before. Before I knew it, I had a little classroom section set up in my house with Mathematics manipulatives, phonics charts, sight-word flashcards and a whiteboard to match along with everything I thought could help me with lesson creation. Essentially, I brought a little classroom into my home so that the learners could have a bit of our classroom in their homes via WhatsApp.

Teaching from home during lockdown became more fun. I had more time to focus on finding ways to teach effectively and less time focusing on admin. I spent hours creating videos, PowerPoint presentations and listening to learners read via WhatsApp voice notes to make sure they were still on track. Reading and comprehension remain the biggest academic struggle I face as a teacher.

WhatsApp was my saving grace during the lockdown. It was the only way I could communicate with my learners and their parents. Everything I did and wanted to do with my learners had to be done via WhatsApp. I have to admit, I felt despondent on numerous occasions when I saw the many different ways that schools with resources were going about online teaching using platforms like Zoom and Google Classroom. And yet, the fact that I was in a context where those kinds of technologies were not realistic options motivated me to work even harder to get through to my learners. I only had WhatsApp, but I had to make it work.

The 'new normal' was starting to feel a bit more bearable, but then reality crept up on me and burst my bubble a few times a day. I go back to feeling stressed about whether my learners were safe, fed, coping, are getting enough gross and fine motor stimulation at home. More importantly, I worried about whether they were all being loved.

Being a teacher in a community where poverty is real made teaching a lot more challenging. I did not have a contact number for every child in my classroom as not every parent has a cell phone. I have learners who do not get academic support at home. I have learners who are left to their own devices and who only find structure and routine at school and in the classroom. "What would happen to them during the lockdown period, and how would they cope in the classroom when they do eventually return?" These kinds of questions sent my anxiety through the roof.

Teaching under lockdown was very difficult as well. I could not actively monitor the learners like I would in a live classroom. I had to teach the parents how to teach their children and at times it became very frustrating for both of us.

The first few weeks back at school were hard. Attendance was poor, the learners and staff were on edge, and I felt like I did not know what I was doing. Eventually, I started finding my feet and the learners started opening up more and then, just like that, schools had to close again. Even more days were lost, and I felt defeated.

When we eventually returned to school, we once again taught so hard. Everyone jumped in. We used every teaching method under the sun to help our learners get ready for their assessments with the little time that we had left. We had to remember to sanitise; we had to remind them about social distancing; we had to adjust to teaching with a mask on without passing out; on top of that, we had to deal with all the administration thrown at us. We did all these things while trying not to lose our minds. On our outside, you could swear we were okay, when in fact, we were a pin needle close to a mental breakdown every single day.

I have to say that my hard work during lockdown teaching paid off. The learners who came to school were at an academic level that I was happy with. All those hours I spent on WhatsApp were worth it. I really expected the absolute worst when they returned, given the amount of contact time that was lost, but I was happy and proud of them and their parents for making sure that they did what was expected of them.

The cherry on top was that I could revisit the resources I had made because my school has interactive whiteboards. These resources served as revision and consolidation. The learners latched on to the content easily because they were already familiar with it. I was also able to work with those learners who had no access to WhatsApp, and they caught up relatively quickly because of the resources we had at the school. This made me realise that we have a very long way to go when it comes to the availability of technology at all schools. If more schools had access to technology, teaching during lockdown would have been so much easier and more bearable.

The lockdown has taught me a lot. It has taught me, personally, to stop trying to be in control and embrace change more. It has also reminded me that my job is one of the most important and serious occupations in the world, regardless of what others may think. The most telling thing is that this pandemic has proven is that our education system is not as effective as it could be and as effective as many think it is. It is too condensed; so much content was removed from the curriculum once we returned to school, yet teachers were still struggling to cover everything, which clearly is a red flag. We have a lot of damage control to do in the coming years.

There were a few positive outcomes. I started opening up to people more, whereas before, I would normally keep to myself and always have my guard up. I learnt to stop doubting my capabilities as a teacher. Gaining this extra confidence really helped improve my mental health, which was negatively affected by the pandemic.

The biggest thing that lockdown teaching taught me was that I am a strong individual. I did the best that I could with what I had, which was not very much to begin with. I did what I was called to do, which is to teach, and I did it well! It reminded me that in this profession, you cannot afford to be lazy. You need to stay on top of the latest technologies, research, and methods so that if something as unexpected as a pandemic happens, you are equipped with an arsenal to face it.

Lastly, teaching during lockdown proved, once again, that teachers are amazing and no matter what is thrown at us, we always come out strong and that is exactly what we did.

4.8   Parents, Parent teachers

> "In the past, I underestimated the power of trust and connection between the school and the home."

AMANDA*
Undisclosed school (Western Cape)*

Due to comorbidities, I had to teach from home. I collected my DBE workbooks from school for the parents to collect from my house. I also prepared worksheets, photocopied at school, and made books for collection. Parents collected these materials between 13:00 to 16:00. Parents were stressed and could not pay attention to working with their children. Many parents, in fact, complained about the daily activities I sent via WhatsApp. The activities were sent to us by our department's curriculum advisors.

I am fortunate enough to have Wi-Fi. This enabled me to download and send information to the learners and the parents. This is not the first year I have a WhatsApp group with my parents. Every year I make use of this platform to share school information, photos, projects, amongst others, with my parents. This year, however, I did not have all the parents telephone numbers to add to the WhatsApp group. Some parents had old numbers while others removed themselves from the group due to low data and a few numbers did not work.

In the beginning, some learners worked in their blue DBE books and took pictures to show their work. Only a few completed their assigned work per day. The workbooks were fun in the beginning, but the children and parents lost interest in schoolwork as the stress levels of job losses, fear, death, and hunger became a reality. The parents responded less and less to the group, and I suspect they made use of the mute functionality. I communicated with parents privately to try and increase responses to the group. This attempt was unsuccessful as well. At most, three parents responded.

Not all children could access the Internet, print booklets, or be on the phone to respond. It was a waiting game to see if there was a response or anything to help and assist parents and learners. I could sense the stress and anxiety of the parents increase due to the unknown. At this stage, educating their children was not a priority. However, I carried on as normal, updating the parent WhatsApp group and the foundation phase teacher's group. Every morning, I would share the WhatsApp group with the Scottsville community group to reach more parents.

Our curriculum advisor updated us with lesson plans for the Grade R to Grade 7 learners. My husband is also a teacher; he received worksheets from various WhatsApp groups. As a collective, we shared all the resources we had with those parents and teachers with whom we had contact. Numerous teachers do not have access to the Internet apart from their handheld devices. I could sense the appreciation from these individuals. The zero-rated websites were welcomed as well as the radio broadcast teachings and the televised programmes.

Teaching during this time was a bit of a hit and run affair. No specific targets could be met, and no follow-up sessions were arranged to establish what the learners had actually done. It was more of a case of praying and hoping for the best. I remained hopeful that the learners would do the work with somebody using the correct methodology to explain the work. I could only hope that the key concepts were understood, and that revision was done. I felt lost during this time, not knowing exactly how to reach my children effectively. I did not like the teaching from a distance as it was beyond my control.

I knew there could not be effective teaching without reliable connections with parents and learners. At home, parents struggled with no internet, no data, no laptops, or even phones compatible with downloading files, links, etc. Teaching online was difficult for me.

During this time, we, as departmental heads, received online training to make use of MS Teams. This training was a struggle. There was an attempt to have conferences and training sessions via MS Teams. Reality check. As older teachers, we are not clued up on the new technologies or very computer literate. I struggled to mute myself, switch on my video and enable my microphones. Thinking back, it sounds comical but not at the time. Sometimes I thought my 21st-century Grade 2 learners would be more capable with a laptop. If only they were around to give me assistance like I would assist them at school.

In class, I feel at home. I am more at ease with observing whether or not learners grasp the work. I am good at planning follow-up lessons around their understanding of a concept. Lessons are pitched at just about the right level to continue with the integration of the next concept. I had a few learners whose level of comprehension was great. They grasp concepts quickly, especially your brainiacs. Covering the curriculum was my main goal. This is the total opposite of teaching from home. Home-schooling leaves you with more questions than answers and a lot of uncertainty.

The ever-changing teaching plans were confusing. It was supposed to be a trimmed curriculum but ended up being more work to be done. Lessons had to be prepared and typed. It was stressful. The curriculum advisors and provincial officials did not have clear directives for the curriculum. In addition, the requirement of having learners at school for only two or three times a week was not a good one.

I did not manage to cover the curriculum as there was a misunderstanding when the Grade 2s went back to Term 3. They started with Term 3 work, but did not cover Term 2's curriculum adequately. There is no way you can build new concepts on an unstable foundation; it is impossible. I believe Grade 2 is one of the utmost important grades. It rectifies Grade 1 and prepares the learner for Grade 3 with concepts built on their existing understanding. However, my hands were tied, I was at home due to comorbidities.

At school, our principal thought it is best to do Term 3's curriculum instead of Term 2. I was instructed to cease communication with the staff as I was on leave. My special Covid-19 leave was subsequently changed to incapacity leave.

At that moment, I felt unappreciated as a teacher and a departmental head. I found the courage to voice my opinion to the circuit manager after one of the Minister of Education's speeches. There was never a time in my life when I felt more disturbed and disappointed being a teacher. I felt like resigning, giving a minute's notice and never to teach again.

Despite the hurt, I stayed positive. The communication I had with my learners and parents encouraged me. I enjoyed direct chats, voice notes and pictures of their work. The interaction I had with them emotionally strengthened the bonds far more than the work that had to be done. We shared prayer requests for families and alike. This time, I managed to encourage my parents with God's word and prayed for them when they collected the workbooks.

Leanne Mahoney
Beaumont Primary School (Western Cape)

I am a Grade 3 teacher at Beaumont Primary School in Somerset West. I have been teaching for over 20 years. Initially, I enjoyed teaching under lockdown. Actually, it was more like *planning* than teaching. I did very little standing-in-front-of-the-class teaching. Instead, I prepared lessons. I made worksheets and activities. I wrote stories and comprehensions. I put together PowerPoints, and I made videos. This work was then sent to the parents via WhatsApp and later was posted onto a Microsoft platform for the parents to access.

Once sent, I then interacted with my class by responding to questions via WhatsApp, or I made quick little explanatory videos. Once a week, I had a Zoom call with my class. About 80% of the children showed up each time, and I chatted to them and gave each child a chance to tell me about something they had experienced that week. It was very informal, but it was a great way for me to see my class and for them to see each other.

That is the short answer. However, there was much more to it.

Since I hardly saw my class face-to-face, I did almost all this work in my pyjamas or my workout clothes. I do not think I wore jeans or a nice shirt for three months! In fact, even when I Zoomed with my class, I was always in my running kit.

I loved my new daily routine. I woke up around 09:00, sat up in bed or at the kitchen counter in my gown and slippers with my breakfast, coffee and laptop. I did my schoolwork until I felt it was time to change into actual clothing. This was any time between 10:00 and lunchtime. I then put on my running clothes and continued with schoolwork on and off for the rest of the day. In between these activities, I managed to do some sweeping, preparing meals, cleaning and running around after a husband, four children, three dogs and a couple of foster kittens.

At 17:00, I jumped on the treadmill. The family knew this was my sacred time, and I got to spend the better part of an hour watching a Netflix show while running nowhere. At 18:00, it was time for dinner and the whole family would sit down to share a meal. This is something which I could never manage to do properly before lockdown with all of our different schedules, sports, homework and other commitments. I was grateful for the small changes. After dinner, once the kitchen was cleaned again, I continued working. I was making a few educational videos at this time for the WCED, so I really needed a quiet time to do this.

My youngest son went to bed, the teenagers either went out to the garage to play table tennis or put on their headphones and became completely antisocial. My husband spaced out in front of the news or a movie. I often worked until after midnight. But of course, it did not matter – I only had to open my eyes again the next morning at nine.

The hardest part for me personally was actually schooling my own children. Luckily my teenage daughters are independent and studious enough to work hard on their own. But my ten-year-old son was a bit of a challenge. His teacher definitely did a better job than I did.

Back at school, I knew parents struggled to teach their children during lockdown. I could certainly see the results of this when we went back to school. Writing skills, handwriting, reading and times tables had taken a serious knock! It took quite some time to get the learners out of some of the bad habits they had developed at home. Many children had not read regularly, even though I spent hours typing out the readers and scanning in pictures. They had not been writing neatly – many had been allowed to simply write answers down any way they liked, without spelling or punctuation rules being followed. Even after all this time, I still feel that reading skills in both their first language of English and the additional language of Afrikaans are not at the usual standard.

I am relieved that we are now back at school. I missed my class, and I really missed actually teaching. However, it is quite different. With only 16 in a class now, I feel as though I am teaching at a private school. We have two sessions each day. The children in the first session arrive any time from 07:00. Officially class starts at 07:50. The learners leave school at 11:00 and the second session begins shortly thereafter. We normally go home around 15:00. It is a much longer teaching day, although, without sport to coach in the afternoons, I am usually home much earlier than before lockdown.

Since the children often arrive at my classroom before school officially starts, I have had to find ways to keep them busy at their desks. I have a PowerPoint saved on my desktop, which I project onto the screen each morning. There is a new slide for each day of the week, and it has tasks for the children to do. As the children arrive in class, once they have sanitised their hands and had their temperatures taken, they sit at their desks and take out their whiteboards and a whiteboard marker. They then follow the instructions on the screen. They may have to count in multiples of 3, 4 or 5, or count in 30-minute increments. There might be a Maths pyramid on the screen or a sudoku puzzle. Sometimes I have typed up a sentence, and the children have to identify the parts of speech. Some days I have shown short video clips or songs. This time is so valuable. Children in the class get the chance to chat to each other and to me before the work of the day actually starts – and they get to improve important academic skills.

When we started this new system in June, when the schools first opened, it was exhausting. I think I went to bed at about 20:00 on the first Friday – even though I had only been at school for three days! Teaching the first session was fine, but it was quite hard teaching the same thing all over again for the second session. It was also so intense. I was extremely aware of the fact that my six hours of contact time each day had been cut in half. I had to make sure that when I taught a concept, it was taught as thoroughly as possible. Of course, the smaller class helped me identify very quickly which learner needed help with which concept. This meant that while my learners were completing tasks, I could zip around the whole class and identify children who needed a little more practice or individual help. I do not think I sat down at my desk for the first three months that we were back. I was so busy marking work and checking on my learners' progress during class time. I would whiz around the class with my red or purple pen, marking and checking and correcting. Now the routine is working perfectly. We have a good rhythm going. Each group is different, so I do not get bored teaching the second session.

The best is that I have occasionally been bringing my foster kittens to school (do not tell my boss!). I was given two little five-week-old kittens to take care of, but with my long workday, I did not want to leave them unsupervised for so long. I created a little den in my old reading corner and kept the kittens in there. Initially, the kittens just stayed there, and I saw to all their needs. However, as time went on, the children and the kittens became bolder. The children – some of whom had never touched a kitten before – started stroking and holding them or letting them play on their desks. Now, if the child has finished their work, they go to the kitten corner and either play with a kitten or take it back to their desk where the kitten falls asleep, tucked into a jersey, or curled up on a lap.

All in all, we are coping in this new situation. We have covered the curriculum in Maths, English Home Language and Afrikaans First Additional Language. We have given a small amount of time to Life Skills. We are teaching much smarter, using one book for all subjects instead of wasting time taking out a different book for each lesson, working off the screen instead of cutting out and sticking in worksheets.

There are two main concerns I have. Firstly, due to time constraints, as well as the social distancing factor, we cannot do group work. There just isn't time for reading groups in the two languages, where I get to explain the book, ask questions, develop comprehension skills, improve vocabulary and improve reading skills. I also cannot have my learners in ability groups sitting on the carpet, solving maths problems together or discussing methods.

Secondly, we have to rely on the parents to ensure that children do their homework. Before lockdown, I had plenty of time to drill times tables, spelling and so on. Now, all that has to happen at home as homework as there really is no time in class. This means that some children are at a disadvantage because they do not do the homework. Some parents struggle to access the homework. We post homework sheets onto the Microsoft platform, as well as the readers and Life Skills tasks, yet parents struggled. Others just do not think it is important enough to make time for reading or learn spelling words. Some also do not understand the importance of learning times tables, or they just leave it up to their children to learn on their own. Children actually need clear guidance and someone to help them to practise.

I honestly hope we never have to experience this again, even though I have learnt a lot and my teaching has improved over this time. We now need to focus on what is important to ensure excellence in education. Face-to-face teaching is vital. We do not need each child to have a fancy tablet – each child needs the basic resources of books and pencils, a safe place in which to learn and have a caring, enthusiastic teacher. Maybe after all this, education in South Africa will improve.

Maryna Sliers
Berzelia Primary School (Western Cape)

Lockdown and isolation, words synonymous with 'solitary confinement'. A phrase generally used in prison, not in schools. Yet, we have started to use these words as if they form part of our everyday vocabulary. Our learners are used to them as well. We heard and read about the 1918 flu pandemic and the destruction it caused, but never did we contemplate a pandemic in our lifetime.

As a teacher, you often hear of the prominent roles we play in our learners' lives: planner, manager, therapist, parent, and friend. But I am also a parent to my beautiful eight-year-old daughter as well as my three-year-old son; in this lockdown, my daughter has also suffered.

Teaching under 'solitary confinement' has had detrimental effects and caused a significant change to our normal daily routine. What do you do when there are only 10-15 learners in your class, and the other 40 are at home? Do you teach? Yes, you do. You know that your learners at home are at a disadvantage. They received their work-from-home packages, but if the parents do not understand the curriculum content, how did we come to expect them to convey it to our learners?

I applaud the government for the extraordinary measures that were put in place to assist our children. But the contexts for learning are still very challenging. I live in a community that's riddled with socio-economic problems, where our learners do not have access to computers, data, etc. And yet, we have to make the best of it. Many of our parents tried really hard to assist their children in learning from home.

I remember how overwhelmed we felt as teachers as we anticipated the return of our Grade 7s. They had been at home for over three months, their longest 'holiday' ever. We only had one child at school on the first day. Our parents were protesting as they felt that our learners' lives were put in danger. The protests continued for about a week until parents were given the option to keep their children at home if that was what they wanted. A lot of parents came to sign for that option. That meant fewer learners in a class, more of them at home.

The school communicated with parents via letters, WhatsApp group, etc. Although not every parent was reached in these ways, we tried. Many parents also complained that neither they nor the child understood the work given to them. That also became worrying for me, as a teacher, because we know the learners will be assessed at the end of the day. How can you assess a learner that you never taught? But that is where our amended assessment plans and -curriculum came in. The curriculum had been adjusted to ensure that the fundamentals had been covered and assessed. With the gradual lifting of the lockdown levels, things improved. As more learners returned, we approached full capacity. Although the time was limited, I stood firm in my role as educator and did what I could under the circumstances.

As a teacher and parent, I know that the 2020 school year will have a long-term effect on our learners' outcomes in future years. Although the fundamentals were taught, we know that difficult years lie ahead.

My daughter is a true testament to this detrimental year. Where should I start? Meghan is eight years old, attending Grade 2 in a public school. Her mother is a language teacher. Meghan is the kind of daughter that will make you happy and angry at the same time. I love her dearly, but I have to admit she is as lazy as can be. She has a natural touch for Mathematics and achieves average to above-average marks in all of her subjects. Sounds like the normal, average child in South Africa, right?

You might also think that Meghan holds an advantage because her mother is a teacher. No, not at all. There were difficult times, still are. Financially and spiritually, in all facets of life. In any event, with the lockdown, Meghan had also received her work-from-home packages at school and had to complete those assignments with the help of a parent or any adult in her life. As a teacher, you would think I would have patience with my daughter, but man, was it difficult. With all of the distractions at home, do not mention her brother who would just randomly come and grab a page, the dog that would come and jump on her, the TV playing her favourite cartoon, and everyone walking up and down because no one would settle down to work.

Meghan being a lazy child, I would give up after, say, an hour. Then her grandparents would take over. My motherly instincts tell me that Meghan is a clever girl that can work independently. I was sure that she was still on par with her work even though she did not complete all her activities.

When the time came for the Grade 2s to go back, I decided to keep her at home. That is hypocrisy, right? I expect parents to send their children to school, but I keep my child at home. Of course, I knew that all safety measures were put in place to ensure her safety, but I was split in two. On the one hand, I am a caring parent who wants to ensure the safety of my child; on the other hand, I am a teacher of more than 100 children who wants to ensure that they have a solid education at school.

After about two weeks, I decided to send Meghan back to school, not just because Meghan was sending my mother to an early grave, but because I could sense that she was not in any way excelling at home. She had also rotated and went to school for two to three days a week. When her third term report card came, Meghan, the above-average child, had performed below-average. She had now gone from Codes 7s and 6s to Code 3s. She failed her subject, Home Language, and as a language teacher myself, I found this unacceptable.

I am a teacher who is a parent whose child had now failed the third term because she was not at school, and I did not do enough to ensure that she stayed on par. I apologised to her, as I had failed her. As teachers, we often forget to take care of ourselves and our loved ones as we spend much more time on work. This year has made it even more difficult. I was so bound by the needs of others that I forgot about my own. If Meghan, an above-average child in South Africa, with the advantage of having a teacher-mother, dropped in her academic achievements, what would happen to less fortunate children in our country?

NADIA WILLIAMS
Matroosfontein Primary School (Western Cape)

Boy oh boy, where do I start? I do not think anything could have prepared us for a pandemic that literally brought the whole world to a stop. I am a novice teacher, teaching in a diverse, multilingual school in Matroosfontein. Most of the learners come from a poor background. Poverty, unemployment, and social problems are rife. Here people live to survive, and many of our learners are on the school's feeding scheme.

I want to share my lockdown experience as a teacher with you, and how I had to work to overcome my own anxiety. Teaching under lockdown was scary. Going out for the first time felt like something out of a movie. For me, the anxious moment was going to pick up groceries. All this seems like a distant memory now.

We were all in the same boat, regardless of background or occupation. It was ten times worse for me as a teacher, mother, and wife. As a teacher, it started kicking in with what this might mean for me and my learners. After all, my school is situated in an area that is very much classified as 'high risk'. I had much anxiety because of where I was based, but the work had to go on. I was very concerned as to when the school would reopen and how we would manage the assessments. How would we cover all the work? What will happen to the rest of the year?

I made contact with my learners' parents through WhatsApp and formed a WhatsApp group. I decided to give extra lessons. This was extremely intimidating. At first, I just forwarded worksheets to parents and learners for them to complete. The parents would be the channel through which to reach my learners. I admittedly did not get many responses from parents at first.

With the help of colleagues, I decided to conduct proper online lessons because I did not feel I was reaching my learners or their parents by just sending out worksheets. I then converted the one side of my bedroom wall into a whiteboard by taking blank paper and covering it with plastic. I started recording myself and started drawing up a lesson plan to work from. As intimidating as it was to do a video lesson, I pushed through. I had set times. I would wake up and try and get the video out by 09:00. This was often quite time-consuming. I would record the video, but it always ended up being too long to send via WhatsApp. Technology can be very challenging at times. I remember trying so many converters to finally convert and compress the video so that it could be sent via WhatsApp.

Finally, I managed to send a video lesson. My video would consist of Maths, First Additional Language (FAL), and Home Language. I would do two videos a day, as I was very mindful of the potential data costs for the parents.

Since 2019, I have belonged to a group called the Primary Science Programme (PSP). This is such a wonderful support group for novice teachers. I was fortunate to have such great support from my mentor, Ms Florence, as well as my school principal, Ms L. Philander, throughout the lockdown. I was never afraid to ask for extra support or advice, which really helped my teaching. They were very supportive and willing to go over the videos the night before and offer new insights to improve the quality of my presentations.

Online lessons were great. Parents and learners started responding. They even asked me for assistance in other areas. It really was a great way to get the parents involved. As I became more comfortable with the technology and the parents, I started moving to PowerPoint lessons. This was awesome, especially for the Maths lessons. While I am no expert, I could see that both the learners and parents started responding positively.

During the lockdown, I also had regular online meetings with parents who were available. I asked my mentor, Ms Florence, to attend the first such meeting. There were only four parents who attended. While I was very disappointed with the low turnout, I persevered. As I progressed with the online technology, I eventually had ten parents showing up. This was big progress, given that these online platforms were new to many parents. I decided to see the glass half full rather than empty.

I had to closely follow a lesson plan to guide my online teaching. The Department of Education also started sending online resources and lessons for us to use and send to the parents. If I've never admitted that I love the Department of Education, I sure did at the time. I absolutely loved using the General Education and Training (GET) lesson plans.

It came with such nice videos, as well as resources. I started working from there and prepared my own videos accordingly. This is where I got the idea to deliver my online lessons using PowerPoint.

I believe that the foundation of parents' willingness to trust in me as a teacher was set during these early days of the lockdown. In preparation for their return to school, I made desk screens for my learners so that they and their parents could feel safer. I also ensured them that I would defog my class at my own cost. Parents in turn showed their support by sending masks and shields. Those gestures meant a lot to me.

When we returned to school, my colleagues and I started making advanced copies of all the worksheets that we would require for each specific lesson. Once we went through the amended curriculum from the department, it was easier to navigate what needed to be done. We also made comprehensions and other booklets ahead of time. We knew it would soon be a 'crunch' time. As a team and a school, we decided that we would concentrate on reading, phonics, and maths in the limited time available

It is so easy to panic and stress about what we cannot control. However, I was blessed to have supportive colleagues in my grade and supportive people in my life to help me get through the year. I firmly believe that this was the only way we managed to cover the curriculum. I have to admit that planning really made a world of difference, especially since we used the GET band lesson plans provided by the department. Despite all the stress and anxiety, I believe that we did well in 2020.

Mariaan Bester
Hillcrest Secondary School (Western Cape)

In April 2020, I was appointed in a teaching position at Hillcrest Secondary School. Lockdown level 5 was in full swing. Prior to this appointment, I was a subject advisor for Physical Sciences and Natural Sciences. There I was with lots of enthusiasm and ready to start teaching. Except the schools were closed, and I would not have an opportunity to meet my new learners.

I created a WhatsApp group for Grade 9 and was amazed at the rate at which the message spread, and the learners joined. I made videos about Mathematics lessons and a daily recognition poster where I acknowledged the learners that send me the homework that I assigned on the WhatsApp group.

The majority of Hillcrest learners come from low- to no-income households. Many of them did not have their own cell phones and connected to the group via their parent's phones. This, I later realised, was a huge plus. More and more parents started to get involved and inquired about their children's learning. Strong partnerships formed between teacher and parents. In the past, I underestimated the power of trust and connection between the school and the home.

I had about 106 learners who regularly received video lessons. About 12 to 15 learners replied daily and sent back their homework. For many teachers, this would be a devastating return on investment. For me, it was a perfect opportunity. In truth, I did not have the capacity to pay individual attention to 106 learners online. I had not yet mastered the skills necessary to explain Mathematics using WhatsApp as a medium. The small but steady stream of learners provided me with just enough feedback to get an understanding of learner context and the opportunity to master appropriate tech skills.

The learner had to choose to engage with me. There were no bells and timetables that forced us into each other's company. Secondly, when (s)he was bored, nothing prevented that learner from leaving the group or walking away from teaching. As a teacher, I had to earn the learner's attention. It was simply wonderful to experience the gratitude, excitement and understanding of learners when things did not go as well as planned.

Besides teaching Mathematics and Science content, the social media experience gave me a golden opportunity to demonstrate and address important skills that are never mentioned in the current curriculum. Many teachers are hesitant to allow learners the freedom to participate in public conversations. As a teacher, one has very little control over things said in the chatrooms. To complicate matters further, many parents also had access to chatrooms. Being vulnerable and exposed to learner behaviour in the presence of an adult audience was daunting. It never occurred to me that it would not only be learners' behaviour that had the potential to be problematic. Apart from spreading fake news, parents periodically posted inappropriate materials.

To me, this was a whole new education stage with loads of new opportunities for doing what I do best: TEACH. So, we addressed issues such as fake news and posting negative or personal comments on a WhatsApp group. We talked about how to develop and maintain a positive ethos in the social media space, what to post, and what not to put out there, etc. I could not always tell if the person reading my post was an adult or a child reading the message. This forced me to treat everybody as adults – with courtesy, respect and most importantly, always using a pleasant tone. This had a tremendous impact on the way that learners treated me.

When we finally returned to school, I soon realised my experience of teaching had completely shifted. The classroom was now an impersonal space, where I struggled to identify learners behind masks. I could not interpret facial expressions or always hear what learners answered in muffled voices. Emojis, voice notes, checking status updates became the space in which I made personal contact and connections with my learners.

In the past, cell phones in class were forbidden. Now I encourage learners to videotape lessons – especially since I did not have enough time to produce enough content videos. Besides feeling like a movie star under constant paparazzi surveillance, I was intrigued by how some over-energetic-unable-to-sit-still-ADHD ping pong balls managed to sit perfectly still, completely focused on videotaping me as I was teaching.

Lockdown brought new rules, new challenges. Ready or not, both learners and teachers were forced to develop critical thinking and problem-solving skills. In the past, it was a well-known fact that learner behaviour became much more problematic when they did not wear school uniform. Now learners were regularly allowed to come to school wearing their normal clothes, and that allowance did not contribute to disciplinary problems. It was an eye-opener to see that some of our beliefs were really outdated or misinformed. The focus changed completely from trying to be the perfect teacher in the perfect teaching environment to being the resilient teacher in challenging and imperfect times.

This was the best and the worst year in teaching. Teaching was brought to a standstill and, at the same time, elevated to a completely new level. Lockdown simultaneously widened the gap between the technological 'haves' and the 'have nots'. The classroom was now the levelling experience for both affluent schools and struggling schools were only allowed to have a smaller number of learners.

My retired friend often sighs, relieved that she is just so glad she does not teach at the moment. I do not think I agree. In many ways, this was the best year in my teaching career, though one I hope never to repeat.

ANGELO ADAMS
Rylands High School (Western Cape)

March 2020 feels like decades ago, that moment when we started living under lockdown conditions, confined to our own homes. The previous month, February 2020, my wife give birth to our first child; those few days being at home adapting to what was going to be our new lifestyle, having to look after and care for our bundle of joy, was amazing. Then I went back to school to wrap up Term 1 and amidst all the nappy changes, burping, bathing and making sure my wife was comfortable as a first-time mother, there were murmurs of a lockdown on the horizon.

At first, I was excited for my own selfish reasons. I looked forward to the prospect of watching my daughter develop while we teachers were on an extended break. I forgot about the responsibilities I had to 1 000 learners at my high school. Soon it dawned on me that my matric group needed me the most. My subject colleague retired in April 2020.

Since we shared the grade as the two senior teachers, the entire matric class became my responsibility, all 205 learners.

Some would say that it was a bit much, but I believe the experience made me a better human being and teacher. The learners were incredible. I created a database of 205 learners. Once established, I managed to convince them that we could complete the syllabus and be ready for the examinations. My focus was automatically set on their finals. Work had to be completed. We had curriculum guidelines. I know the syllabus back to front, and it was unlikely that much would change.

The only challenge I faced was getting each learner to subscribe to my new method of teaching. I sent voice notes, video clips, infographics, resources overloaded, past exam papers and worked overtime, getting them ready for their exams. They took to it like ducks to water and made the transition effortlessly. One or two difficulties arose but sending data was such a simple task. We created a sense of responsibility amongst us as a group. We were accountable to each other, and when we finally got back to school, we could engage in person like old times, albeit behind masks and an abundance of sanitiser.

Teaching became repetitive once we got back to school, smaller classes but more of the same. The learners with comorbidities needed extra support, and that is where hybrid learning became my new reality. I would teach at school but also teach for an hour or two once at home. All this while juggling parenting, responding to messages and emails from parents, and supporting learners at almost any hour of the day or night.

Whether the 2020 academic year could be considered a success has yet to be seen. The success we could witness was in how young people proved how easy It was for them to adapt to a new way of living and learning in pandemic times. I hope and pray that these young people will always remember their fight, grit and determination to make 2020 one for the books.

Astrid Adams
The Hague Primary (Western Cape)

Teaching under lockdown has been challenging. When I first heard the news in March 2020 that our country was going into hard lockdown, I was so unprepared. I had none of the parents' numbers on my phone because I stored it all in a file at school. I did not think I would need it because I did not understand at the time what lockdown meant. I also preferred to keep my number private as I have a history with parents who struggled with boundaries. As a result, there was no communication with parents in what became an extended holiday.

As soon as I returned to school (May 2020), I created a parent communication WhatsApp group that at least connected to some of the parents. The reality of teaching in a disadvantaged community on the Cape Flats is that not all parents have a cell phone, while some had phones that could not WhatsApp. This meant that doing WhatsApp lessons or sending electronic notes was out of the question. I found myself copying notes and asking parents to collect it every second week for the other grades while I was teaching all the Grade 7s Creative Arts at school.

I found that parents were also scared of contracting the virus. Some did not even care to collect the notes I prepared diligently for two months. By the time my Grade 5 learners returned in August/September, many of them had not done any schoolwork for the last five months. I knew instantly there was a lot of repairing I had to do. I teach Mathematics to all four Grade 5 classes. I had to find a way of making the most of the contact time with each group which came to about 19/20 days for the term. Children were divided into two groups that attended school on alternate days.

I prepared a set of notes that the learners received on the so-called "orientation days", which was the first two days back at school after lockdown. Parents who applied for their children to do home-schooling could also come and collect the prepared notes that covered the term's work. Usually, I would write the notes on the board and explain it afterwards, but this was out of the question because of the limited time we had with the returning children. I requested the learners to write the notes at home on their 'off-days' so that on their days at school, I would explain the content to them. This arrangement allowed for more time for one-to-one teaching.

Somehow, I managed to fit in the work from Terms 2 and 3 in a short period. I had to catch up with Term 2's work because many learners did not get the notes and I knew that parents would struggle to teach the curriculum to their children because many of them did not complete school themselves.

Absenteeism was a challenge. I had to constantly phone and send letters home to parents of learners who did not want to come to school. This meant more 'admin' and we already had extra administration to contend with. Most time, I had about 90-100% school attendance. During this time, some of my learners lost parents or other family members due to the virus. It was a very difficult time and I had to comfort these learners as best I could, offering them support with soft and gentle words.

At the end of Term 3, we had to complete an assessment for Mathematics. I saw a massive change in the results. Many of the learners did better because of the grouping system. The smaller classes allowed for one-to-one teaching, which saw many of the learners excel in Mathematics. Learners were eager to participate in these smaller classes. They seemed to grasp more complex concepts. My weaker learners now did better than those learners who were usually stronger in maths. Learners who stayed absent a lot did poorly because they missed out on teaching time.

I am also thankful that the Department trimmed some of the unnecessary content because this meant the learners and teachers had less pressure to cover a packed curriculum. I could finally cover all the content that the Department expected us to do, using my personal judgement for deciding on the amount of time devoted to each topic.

I could also use this time to reflect and prepare for the final term. By the last day of school, my notes for Term 4 were already made and copied. The learners each received their notes just in case we got another wave of the pandemic and be forced into a hard lockdown again. This time I would not be as unprepared as in the beginning.

4.9 Peer teaching

> "It was simply amazing that teachers I had never spoken to before, more experienced teachers, all came together to help each other."

WEDAAD ESAU
Jamaica Way Primary (Western Cape)

My name is Wedaad Esau and I am a first-grade teacher in Mitchells Plain for seven years. I always start my year with a 'meet the teacher' opportunity where I encourage parents to join my WhatsApp group so that we have a quick and easy way to communicate. This year was no different. I have a diverse class of 40 learners, where not all my learners speak the language of learning, however, 90% of my parents are part of my WhatsApp group and this created good communication from the start.

The announcement in March 2020 that schools would close was a bit overwhelming because the last week of the term is one of my busiest times. I must complete reports, get my 'admin' done, set up a holiday programme, plan a fun activity for the holidays, etc. With the early closure notice, I was not able to do most of these things. However, I was able to set up a two-week holiday programme for my learners. I informed my parents that if they needed any assistance with schoolwork, they would be welcome to contact me.

I felt at ease knowing that my learners had work to keep themselves busy at home and that, when they return, we could start where we left off. Then the unforeseen happened. The country would be going into a 21-day lockdown and school would not be opening as scheduled.

At first, I was not worried because I knew that I would be able to send my learners lessons via WhatsApp. However, I was concerned about how I was going to do my lessons in order to make it easy for my learners and parents to understand, knowing that half of them do not speak English at home. I also wanted them to be able to engage with me so that I knew if they understood what I was teaching. I want it to be fun and practical for parents and learners alike.

I decided to research the best way to teach while at home and still engage my learners. I started to watch YouTube and found that many teachers around the world had the same questions. Many educators were doing virtual teaching using various methods to teach, such as Zoom, Google Classroom, ClassDojo, and so many others. I knew this was not an option for me because many of my parents were not able to get access to these apps due to the costs and amount of data they would need.

I started to contact other first grade teachers in the area to find out how they were teaching, which methods they were using, and how they felt about all of this. It was simply amazing that teachers I never spoke to, more experienced teachers, all came together to help each other because we had one goal in mind, and that was to teach well enough so that our learners could understand. We decided to do video lessons which were sent via WhatsApp. The lessons were fun, engaging, and easy to understand.

All parents had to do was let their children watch the lessons and do the activities. I thought this was brilliant, the best solution to the problem we were facing. I did not realise that this plan would cause its own problems. For starters, parents were not able to download the video because it required too much data. Some parents were also still working, and the child was left with siblings. There were also social problems that interfered with learning from home. As a result, I only had 40% of my learners doing the lessons. This was not good enough.

I started to feel frustrated and upset because I was trying to teach and to assist my learners in every way I could. It just was not working out, no matter how hard I tried. I understood that the parents were trying, but their constraints were real and beyond our control. The situation made me feel so helpless.

Just then, we received the WCED e-portal lessons via WhatsApp and I was able to download it and send it to my parents; this worked a little better because I then had 50% of my learners doing the work. However, I was still worried about the learners that I was not able to contact, and those with social problems at home.

I was still sending lessons and chatting to my learners, but I so much wanted to be at school. School is my happy place where I can help my learners in so many ways, not just by teaching them but also being there to encourage and uplift them. Finally, we were able to return. I was ecstatic but still worried since my grade learners were still not back. We set up book packs with work to assist our learners and communicated this to parents.

My biggest regret about the 2020 academic year. Is that I could not be there for all my learners, I could not teach the fun, engaging lessons the way I normally would. I was not able to build a strong relationship with them or help develop the social skills they needed to be competent.

This year parents and teachers improved their communication with each other. An improved level of respect was established, and their roles in the learners' lives acknowledged. Department, unions, and educators all communicated to ensure the best for all parties involved. Teachers around the world came together to build a community of educators in which they found support and encouragement.

JULIE-ANN LENDRUM
Winchester Ridge Primary (Gauteng)

I teach Grade 7 English Home Language in a suburban public school situated in the south of Johannesburg. Our 1 184 learners come from diverse socio-economic and cultural backgrounds. When the initial lockdown began, parents were given a summary of websites and links posted by the DBE to give parents activities to do with their children at home.

When the lockdown was extended, teachers realised that learners were going to miss out on the curriculum. There was much uncertainty as to how this was going to be addressed. Teachers at our school set up their own Google Classrooms for their subjects. Using social media and announcements via the school's D6 Communicator, learners were notified and began logging on. By the end of the lockdown, we had about a 60% attendance of learners on Google Classroom.

This was an exciting time for teachers and learners alike. We were thrust into the world of online teaching and technology. Teachers enjoyed the new learning experience and enjoyed discovering what learning tools and resources exist online. The learners surprised us.

For example, I had the learners complete the submission of their English speech online. They had to video-record the speech on their mobile phones and submit the MP4 file on Google Classroom. YouTube videos were provided on how to take a 'selfie' video and how to make a digital presentation. We were amazed by the response as learners seemed to enjoy this added dimension to their learning. What we did find interesting was the fact that many learners who seemed to be mediocre performers in class performed well online as they enjoyed working with the technology. Their experience of success served as motivation to complete the tasks.

As can be expected, one of the drawbacks of using Google Classroom was the lack of access to data on the part of many socio-economically disadvantaged learners. Many learners and parents also did not have the technical know-how required to access Google Classroom. In addition, not all teachers had the technical training required or have access to data and laptops.

To ensure no learner was left behind, all work done via Google Classroom was repeated in class when schools reopened. Learners who had done the work online simply had to hear it again in class.

When school reopened, Grade 7 classes of 40 learners were divided into two classes of 20 for purposes of social distancing. Initially, the atmosphere was dismal. There was a pall of quiet over the school as learners nervously stood apart from each other with masks covering parts of their faces. Nobody dared to speak, smile, or laugh. The school seemed like a mausoleum. No other Grades were at school. Teachers from other grades pitched in to teach classes alongside the Grade 7 teachers. For example, all intermediate and senior phase English teachers taught Grade 7 English, all Maths teachers taught Maths.

Foundation phase teachers were also given classes to teach relevant to their area of expertise. The learners remained in class and the teachers rotated to ensure that there was minimum movement in the corridors while learners remained at one desk for the entire day. There were several benefits to the new arrangements. The learners were taught their subjects by subject specialists using a variety of teaching styles. The foundation phase teachers, who had never taught higher grades, were able to gain insight into where the foundations that they laid lower done the school system led to. Teachers had 5-10 minutes more in each lesson since masses of learners were not moving around.

While only one grade was at school, teachers of the other grades continued teaching with Google Classroom and help learners who were struggling with the new technologies. Google Classroom was streamlined and made more secure, and each learner was given their own e-mail address. Teachers also prepared learning packs for parents to pick up to continue teaching children at home so that the curriculum could be covered during the lockdown.

When the rest of the grades returned to school, some changes were made. The learners quickly got used to the new situation and once again there was laughter and fun in the corridors.

On their return, it was disappointing to find that even though learners had logged on to Google Classroom or had collected work packs, this work had not been completed at home. This could be due to a lack of expertise on the part of parents or to the fact that there was no supervision at home. I have also found that learning online requires much reading. It appears that reading to learn, especially in the primary school context, has hampered the success of online learning.

Discipline definitely improved with smaller classes. I was able to get through a substantial portion of the curriculum. As an English teacher, I found that my learners were not really disadvantaged as far as curriculum coverage was concerned. A lot of superfluous and repetitive aspects were removed; I liked the new core, streamlined curriculum. I could now reinforce essential content and focus on weaker learners while at the same time stimulating stronger learners.

With 542 of the 1 184 learners attending school each day, there is less of a toll on the resources of the school; at the same time, there was a calmer atmosphere on the school grounds, which in turn was conducive to learning. However, the absence of sport or other extramural activities detracts from the holistic development of the child. We have also not been able to take part in cultural activities like Eisteddfods, public speaking festivals and concerts.

Some learners opted not to return to school and continue learning online at home. This has put an extra toll on teachers who now had to teach a few learners online at home, teach regular classes for those who showed up, provide learning packs for learning from home without online resources, and four classes twice, given the halving of the regular classes per regulation.

On the positive side, teachers have now been exposed to online teaching opportunities, which would not have happened otherwise. YouTube, Google Classroom, PowerPoint, Doodly and similar software provides exciting learning tools that can be incorporated in the course of face-to-face teaching. I admit that I rather enjoyed lockdown teaching with the stimulation and learning it afforded me, and to really get to know my learners and support them.

JADE DAMONSE
Rhodes High School and Soneike High School (Western Cape)

I could never have imagined that in my fifth year of teaching, I would have to start from scratch. By the 23rd of March 2020, learners were already at home and with the lockdown being announced, it just seemed like an extended holiday. However, for my Grade 12s, I knew this could not be the case. I decided that I would start my first lesson on 31 March 2020, as the school calendar stated, as this would have been the first day of Term 2.

Teaching under lockdown took all of me. In my head, it would be this exciting venture, as I would be able to incorporate even more technology into my teaching. I did not, however, realise what this truly meant for me as the teacher as well as the learners.

Let me set the scene. All my lessons for the term were already prepared. The problem was that schools closed sooner than expected, and we would not return on the scheduled date. Even so, teaching had to continue. Not only did I have to redo my planning, but also restructure lessons to suit the current reality.

The reality was that I no longer shared a classroom with my kids. Nor did I have equipment at home and yet learning had to take place. I had no choice but to get smart with technology, and that could only be done by using technology. I watched YouTube videos and attended webinars which enabled me to navigate my way around Facebook, which was my chosen platform for teaching under lockdown.

Teaching online came with its challenges, and the first was ensuring that all my learners had access. I did so by starting a crowdfunding page and, once everyone was online, teaching began. What once seemed like a challenge, turned out to be something I was grateful for. Teaching during lockdown forced me to work with minimal resources, and this was the most significant change in my teaching approach.

The education department was the root of quite a few stressors, as they implemented new changes just as you thought you were getting the hang of things. The main thing for me was to stay calm, to my learners at least, because someone had to provide some sort of stability in the crisis.

I gradually got the hang of Zoom, Loom, and the other platforms we use to teach. I remember how floored I was after my first live lesson on 31 March 2020. "Share screen" was my biggest enemy in the beginning stages of this new way of teaching, and I ended up recording my screen with my cell phone for the first few lessons. It was challenging, but the responsibility that I felt towards my learners is what pushed me to make my page successful. I can honestly say that I have made great strides teaching under lockdown.

Technology is great, but there is nothing that beats the look on a learner's face when they have grasped a concept or even that look when they have not grasped it. Teaching online was so different from teaching in the classroom. In the beginning, learners were too shy to ask questions online. They would later ask their questions privately, which meant that I would be teaching the same lesson or answering the same question more than three times.

I taught via Facebook, as this was the most accessible and affordable platform for my kids. With the Facebook live sessions, you are not able to see the learners, like you would on Zoom; this meant that my probing skills had to be top-notch, as I could not gather from their faces if they were still following or not. This definitely changed how teaching took place, and as time went by, I learnt to put more into the pre-reading section of the lesson to try and eliminate as much confusion or uncertainty as possible.

In terms of coverage, my Grade 12s managed to finish all their poems by the time we returned to school in June 2020. Of course, this content needed to be revised. The setwork proved to be more of a challenge as we did not have enough time to read together during class. This meant that I was not able to pick out words that they did not understand or explain things on the spot. I made a vocabulary list of each of the chapters or Acts and students reported back that they enjoyed being able to read at their own pace. If they did not finish an allocated reading, the learners could on their own time go back to the Facebook page and watch the saved lesson live.

For my other grades, I sent out weekly planners with only one recorded video on a curriculum topic. Effective teaching only happened from mid-April 2020 as teachers and learners started to understand what was expected; this made the online teaching experience much easier. We certainly planned to complete the curriculum for English Home Language assisted by the amendments sent through by the department.

These amendments showed us that there is a lot of unnecessary testing that takes place within the system. Another insight is that we all worked together to provide students with the best resources and teaching experience, something which I had not seen in my five years of teaching. All stakeholders pulled together and did their bit to normalise the disruptions which students had to endure. We also learnt that there really is no need to put so much academic pressure on learners.

About 50% of my learners returned to the classroom, and as the weeks went by, I had more than 80% in my class. I was grateful to have most of them back in the classroom so that I could now show off my newly acquired technology skills.

Through re-designing and restructuring my content, I rediscovered my love and passion for teaching and this is something, which I am grateful to have learnt in the course of the pandemic.

SUNITHA SINGH
Amanzimtoti High (KwaZulu-Natal)

As I think about five to six months of teaching under lockdown, I fervently hope that we never have a repeat of what this year has been like. In about two decades of being an educator, the challenges we were confronted was definitely one for the record books.

Although there were some positives along the way, these were far outweighed by the constant confusion and mental exhaustion that we experienced daily.

For bystanders, it seemed as if teachers were enjoying an extended holiday. This was so far from the truth. The anxiety, uncertainty and responsibilities that accompanied the lockdown cannot adequately be expressed in words.

I missed the interaction with my learners at school. I missed the smiles, the noise, the laughter, those 'lightbulb' moments, the list goes on. I felt disconnected. The digital connection came nowhere close to the connection that we share with our learners daily. I realised at this stage that I took so much for granted. As much as I missed teaching my learners face to face, I realised that I needed to prepare myself to become digitally competent with regards to multimodal ways of teaching. I realised that I needed to go the extra mile and adjust my style of teaching.

I maintained contact with my learners through WhatsApp groups (an idea that I was initially against) and uploaded work on the school's D6 Communicator. The interaction with my learners on WhatsApp made me realise how much I value and respect them. As much as I missed them, liaising with them made me feel that much closer to them in a way and I admire the fact that they really respected my interaction with them. They were grateful for every bit of information received.

I also began to familiarise myself with Google Classroom, and I must admit that it did not come without its challenges. Brushing up on my computer skills was a plus factor for me; I often see myself as technologically challenged. I am part of a resource portal group where the teachers constantly shared resources, designed new and innovative ways of helping learners, and supported each other through the lockdown.

The challenge that I was constantly faced with was whether I was doing enough. Was I able to reach out to all my learners? Did they understand what was required of them? How do I engage learners' interest? As a teacher of English, I constantly asked myself how do I bring a book and characters to life for my learners? How do I make poetry come alive? How do I get learners to engage with a text or poem critically?

My children asleep, I spent most of my nights doing audio recordings to help my struggling learners grasp a better understanding of the novel. My predominant concern at this stage was my Grade 12 learners and whether we would have sufficient time to complete the syllabus in preparation for their National Senior Certificate (NSC) examinations. Now, more than ever before, extensive time was spent on designing lessons for learners who were sitting behind a screen. Often learners did not have data to download resources that I posted on their groups.

Equally challenging for me as a teacher-mom was trying to teach my learners at school whilst trying to home-school my three primary school kids as well. Maintaining the balance became extremely difficult on some days.

I must admit that sometimes just listening to a message tone became exhausting because I knew that might be a learner who needs help. When you are super exhausted, to think of typing long messages or explaining something via a text message could feel overwhelming. My concern was predominantly on how to reach out to learners who did not have cell phones, computers, and internet connectivity. How would they catch up? This was a whole new challenge on its own. I realised that work done during lockdown would have to be re-taught, but the greatest uncertainty was when schools would reopen as Covid infection rates escalated rapidly. At this stage, the reopening of schools seemed further and further away.

Our learners relied on us to give them clarity on when they would be coming back to school, but unfortunately, we too were uncertain about what was happening. As the Covid spread, so did our anxiety. However, I felt that my duty as an educator was to keep my learners calm and let them know that things will get better; yet deep within me, I also had my deep concerns for my own health and that of my family.

I believe that as frontline workers in the education system, our need and support towards each other was greater and came to the fore more than ever before. In the face of adversity, we as educators stood together with the one common denominator being our learners and doing the best we could for them and their futures. The camaraderie between educators was fantastic and the support of the community made us more resilient to handle anything that came our way.

Teaching under lockdown presented me with valuable life lessons and opportunities to reflect on and acknowledge my personal growth along the way. What was once taken for granted is now valued. Teaching under such circumstances forced me to step out of my comfort zone, which I think I still would have been stuck in had it not been for the lockdown. Yes, I was overwhelmed, exhausted and anxious but the one thing that kept me going is that the love for my job.

As I reflect on this time in my life, I am truly grateful that I found new ways to love teaching, even if it meant virtually, I thanked God daily that I had a job! I realised how much I truly loved and missed my learners and, apart from my family, that they too give my life a purpose. Teaching under lockdown offered me a whole new perspective on life. For that, I will always be grateful – grateful that so many individuals surround me daily who impact my life in more ways than I can imagine.

DENE STANFLIET
Berzelia Primary School (Western Cape)

Teaching under lockdown has not been easy. There are rules and safety precautions to follow, and that makes it hard to have the proper one-to-one with learners. The fact is many learners need that one-to-one attention and assistance. The adjustments we had to make were complicated at first, especially when I saw how worried the learners were in the first weeks after they returned to school.

Learners would eventually adapt to the new normal, but there were times they need to be reminded about the safety measures as they have the tendency to forget things such as not sharing with their friends or sitting close to them during break. You have to remind them about wearing masks as well. It was a challenge but we got through it.

The amount of time allocated for teaching and assessments was short but achieved in the end. We had to adjust to the new curriculum, which seemed impossible at first, but once learners were in the classroom, they made it very possible. I had to get used to not being able to sit one-to-one with my learners in my class, and I had to rearrange my class in such a manner that all my learners still got the support from me and their peers; I encouraged peer learning before lockdown.

Meeting the new curriculum requirements of the department was difficult in the beginning but with support from my colleagues, the adjustment was made. My colleagues gave me guidance and support when I needed assistance; this helped me a great deal as many of them have more teaching experience than I do.

We did not have much online teaching. Those parents who could be contacted, made learning from home easier. Some parents showed an interest in their children's education, stayed in communication, and could contact me when they needed guidance.

Teaching students in the class is a better approach for me as I can see in front of me what they are truly struggling with. Some parents had trouble assisting their children and would give their children the answers instead of letting the child do it on their own; this made my task as a teacher more difficult.

I had access to a personal laptop and the Internet. There was also WhatsApp, which is my main tool which I used to communicate with the parents. I had parents who 'video-called' me to explain work they did not understand, just to show them how I would have explained it to the child.

There was not much time for teaching as the learners came back later than expected. There was about half a year of teaching that took place, and that includes the first term. I did not expect to finish much of the curriculum. We would finish about three-quarters of the curriculum for the school year.

The learners were negatively affected by this pandemic. I had learners in my classroom who did not qualify for academic progression due to not receiving the necessary support and teaching. Those learners had to work extra hard to achieve the results that they achieved before lockdown. We also have weak learners who need the one-to-one support. I feel that 2020 really took its toll on some of the learners when it comes to their education and well-being.

Attendance was abysmal to begin with. As the weeks went on, it improved as many parents were at first afraid, but as learners regularly came to school, the word spread about how things were being done, and this made parents more comfortable to be able to send their children to school.

Personally, I have learnt many new things that have helped me improve as a teacher. And I have learnt to face any and all challenges head-on. I also learnt that you should always try your best in everything you do and if you do not get something right immediately, you should always try and try again.

4.10 Perseverance

> "Looking back, I can say that I faced giants and conquered them."

JANIENNE KING
John Ross College (KwaZulu-Natal)

Teaching under lockdown has been a life-changing experience. I teach English Home Language at a school where the mother tongue of children is not English, and the language is not practised at home. Despite that, we do very well academically, and our learners are known for the quality of their English.

We are based in the town of Richards Bay. Nearly all of our learners are disadvantaged. Many live in the nearby townships without both parents, and many have social problems. What distinguishes our children is their spirit, and the fact that we are producing proud, confident, tolerant, open-minded learners who have much to offer South Africa.

When lockdown came, I arranged with one of my learners to make a class group chat on WhatsApp. My school does not have the capacity for online teaching, nor do most of the learners have the capability to receive online. I stayed in constant touch because it was clear to me that many of the learners were afraid and even depressed.

This year one of the matric poems is called *Motho Ke Motho Ka Batho Babang* – a person is a person because of the other people. The notion of Ubuntu is strong in this community. This idea summarises 12NM (the name of my Grade 12 English class) in 2020. We have been a family. We were there for one another and supported one another. Under hard lockdown at home, *Hamlet* was completed, and *Life of Pi* started.

I have been teaching for 35 years, but this year was different. From the moment we came back to school, something special was born. I am a principal and people look to me to be positive and set the tone with 12NM. Every class you teach leaves something of itself with you and shapes you, but 12NM has been extra special. 29 different and unique personalities have made 2020 something noteworthy. From the first day that we returned, we decided to continue the learning process. This process was filled with fun and much more than just English, it was about life.

Not once did the learners complain about Covid, or not having a matric ball or prize-giving. With three weeks to go before finals, we covered the syllabus, except for two poems. We have learnt to write from the heart, we have dissected *Life of Pi*, and we have talked about everything from Black Lives Matter to the Tour de France. We squeezed in some movies just for fun, and Heath Ledger is now hot property in 12NM. We did a quick history of WW2 when we taught 'Vultures' (a poem by Nigerian novelist Chinna Achebe), and we argued about teenage relationships and the generation gap. My class was always about 98% full (the matrics, in general, were about 75% present) and I have learnt so much from them. I have undoubtedly been a better teacher under lockdown because time is so precious.

We had a few cases of Covid and early on the whole school was tested by the Department of Health, who came back later to congratulate John Ross College on the spirit of its students. We were the first school in the area to have a Covid case on return, but we learnt a lot and kept going.

We finished writing trials. We had Grades 8 and 10 one week and Grades 9 and 11 the next week. Our experience has been that they did little work even though we distributed booklets, but they nearly all came to school when it is their turn. It is a sad fact – South African learners lack self-discipline and some saw Covid as a holiday. Many of our learners have teachers for parents, and they will tell you, they do not need to work because they will all pass anyway. How I hope that is not true. Education will be set back by years if it is.

Our learners wear masks with no trouble and are screened and sanitised happily every day. The school sponsored them a mask each and they look smart. Wipes and sanitiser have cost us a small fortune (we are Quintile 5 due to our location), so we got limited help from the Department of Education.

As a principal, I have found that Covid brought out the best in some staff and the worst in others. The genuine fear is noticeable. Some teachers have gone the extra mile. We had no teachers work from home. However, staff solidarity suffered when we had to have two staffrooms. We had superb support from our Superintendent of Education Management, who deserves a medal. The secretarial staff has been tremendous too.

My experience of teaching with Covid has been a blessing. 12NM has never stopped trying. They have offered me hard work, compassion, support, so much joy, and so much love. Knowing that they were looking to me for leadership has given me courage and helped me to be positive in the face of one of the biggest challenges I have ever faced. From the girls who eat all the sweets before trials to the boys who come for calming oil, to the messages I receive every day, these learners are one of a kind.

Some call me Momzy. Yip spelling, I know. One of my favourite moments was when I was told I love you, Mam. Truce bob. And when a pupil told me that his improvement was not enough for the quality of my teaching, you can imagine how humbled I was. This year, under lockdown, I have had 29 children of my own, but more than that, 12NM gave me hope for the future in so many ways.

Lockdown has been a strange kind of blessing. But then, isn't life like that too?

Thea Mendlula
Glenvista High School (Gauteng)

I have never felt as out of my depth as I did during the lockdown period. Not only did I have Grade 12s to worry about but also a group of first-year university students. I was lucky to have established a WhatsApp group with my Grades 11 and 12 learners, and that became the lifeline through which I kept my concerns about their academic progress in check.

On the one hand, I had to familiarise myself with Blackboard Learn and deal with my anxiety about being able to prepare, record and host a group of students via an unknown online platform whilst participating in online tutorials about how to use the platform. Every insecurity I had about my technological skills raised its head. Every single day I had to brush my anxiety aside to reassure my high school group that all is well and that they would not have to repeat the year. My teaching rotated between WhatsApp and Blackboard Learn to the point of extreme exhaustion. I was home but hardly present and remained glued to my laptop.

My recordings for the online platform were done in my car to block out the noise of having three kids, a music-loving husband, and noisy dogs. This did not help me at all but rather turned me into a grumpy pyjama-clad workaholic who hardly ever surfaced other than to tell everyone how insensitive they were to my difficulties. My anxiety before recording my lessons caused diarrhoea and unhealthy snacking. I fell asleep with my laptop, books, marking desk and snacks, while trying to make the most of every day.

I fear to calculate the amount of money we spent on data to keep me connected when our Wi-Fi connection decides to act up and the anxiety of having to switch to my mobile phone. All the while, I sat with the guilt of not doing enough for my matriculants or allaying the fears of the Grade 11 group about what might rob them of a future.

My interaction with the high schoolers centred mainly on reassuring them that we would be prepared for the final examination and that the time lost during the lockdown would easily be recovered. I hardly believed it myself but kept a brave demeanour because, at that stage, hope was all we had. Interacting with my senior learners became a space where we could share an occasional song and memes to bring some sunlight into a clouded reality – that we might not see some of our friends and family again when it is all over. Bob Marley's song 'Three Little Birds' was but one of the few ways I could comfort them. I kept them informed about online platforms which they could use to follow and participate in lessons. I had to remind myself not to overwhelm them with information as it caused unnecessary anxiety. The online connection opened a floodgate of questions which I did not necessarily have time to answer.

Our return to school led to a new level of anxiety because we were all afraid and did not know what to expect. It was one of the most stressful periods of my life. My anxiety-induced asthma started acting up. Despite the cold, the classroom doors had to be left open for ventilation purposes and left me feeling sorry for myself. There was really no way to get around the restrictions brought on by Covid-19.

Our school opted to have our learners redistributed amongst the available teachers, and each of us ended up with different learners to teach! This caused much anxiety amongst our learners as they had to adapt to a new teacher. It was time for us teachers to come up with strategies which made it possible for each teacher to teach the exact same content, so learners did not feel the need to compare or feel as if they received less instruction than their peers. The approach to literature was changed. The novel we read was summarised and compressed into bite-size pieces and distributed to learners via Google Classroom and WhatsApp.

The uncertainty about where and how this will end was one of the things I consciously avoided discussing in class – that was our safe space. The lack of information and differentiated approaches by schools became a bone of contention and comparison amongst teachers. We could feel the anxiety levels rise amongst ourselves. The mutual trust amongst colleagues was strained because we do not know who could possibly be next. This was further fuelled when Grade 12 educators had to return to school and, in addition to their regular teaching, were roped in to fill the gaps where teachers were absent due to comorbidities. It did not help that there were departmental delays with substitute teachers.

What seemed so far off at one stage was right upon us, and it felt all so surreal. Coupled with all the pressure of being able to produce quality passes, many of the School Governing Body-employed educators were informed that their contracts would not be renewed. School principals were able to tick the departmental checklist about the number of things they complied with, but the emotional, physical, and financial losses as a result of lockdown were not confined to job losses in the private sector. Schools sometimes place affordability in respect of human resources above experience and competence. The effect of job losses amongst teachers will ring through the basic education sector for many years to come. In the meantime, all teachers can do is make sure that the learners currently in their care get the best of them.

Looking back, I can say that I faced giants and conquered them.

Dean Skippers
Timour Hall Primary School (Western Cape)

Lockdown teaching during a pandemic brought new and unexpected changes. As educators, we had to embrace the new normal everyone was talking about. We now taught in the absence of 'hot bodies' and not in the familiar, structured classroom. We persevered. As the department altered the syllabus, I transformed my teaching methods too. Teaching Afrikaans and the Natural Sciences, I realised the typical worksheets used every day would not suffice; the D6 Communicator allowed me to upload a variety of resources.

I had to identify the available technologies for effective teaching. I had to consider the socio-economic backgrounds of my learners. I went onto E-Classroom and adapted everything I got my hands onto. WhatsApp groups were created to contact parents effectively. I privately texted learners who were struggling and used the WhatsApp video call facility to explain further and to further illustrate concepts that learners did not grasp the first time.

Online teaching was a formidable challenge as not all parents had phones or data. Instructions that were clear to me were unclear to the parents. Not everything was taught, as I was unsure whether the majority of parents were accessing the information at all. Some parents and learners did not respond to the teachers' communication.

My Grade 4 learners were deeply affected as they spent very little time in school. Even in a normal year, the jump from Grade 3 to Grade 4 is enormous. They needed an educator to guide, assist and show them certain things. When school re-opened, approximately 70% of learners returned. As time went by, the attendance of learners increased.

On returning, things were not the way they were before, for both teacher and learners. The learners were just as overwhelmed as their teachers. From classes of 40, we now have 20 learners in each classroom to comply with the social distancing rules. Learners were encouraged to sanitise as much as possible and to wear a mask at all times.

Teaching under lockdown taught me to tap into my creativity; it led me to adapt, alter and plan thoroughly. Most importantly, it taught me that digital or virtual platforms simply cannot beat the presence of a teacher in the classroom.

4.11 Pastoral care

> "My own anxieties were no longer of any consequence. As a principal, I had to show up and dig deep to be of service to my staff."

PRECIOUS SIPOKAZI GWAYI
Protea Primary School (Eastern Cape)

"Restored to heal the brokenness" is the phrase that carried me to this location. January 2020, in a hidden location of Port Elizabeth, I find myself finally starting my first year as a mainstream teacher. It is not my first year of teaching, but at least this group will be with me from the start of the year until the end, or so I had wished.

I came to Forest Hill, where I assumed duty after fighting the will and direction of my Creator. I decided that He could have only chosen me because I had what it took to influence a child to become more than just academically stable. Little did I know that my sense of normality would end in March. Everything else would be back to basics, a series of endless questions, emotional turmoil, and huge demand to become creative in teaching.

There were so many uncertainties. Individuals posed questions I could not answer. Many felt entitled to denounce teachers and debate our profession. Suddenly it became a profession in the hands of every other profession. It was heartbreaking to witness because we as educators were given a back seat in our own profession.

I occupied the dining table in the morning. I teach all subjects in Grade 5 and isiXhosa to Grades 6 and 7. Somehow, I had to also set papers in both English and Afrikaans. I found myself arranging work for the children while at home in both languages and still provide isiXhosa notes for my isiXhosa groups. That is normal, right?

It was extremely difficult to create content for my isiXhosa groups. I could not trust the language usage of online videos and pictures to get my point across. I cannot quote and make use of overseas resources. I had to find something local. It was important as a teacher to be relevant to current affairs, especially Covid-19. Nothing on the Internet helped with isiXhosa-related work for the intermediate phase. There were no word searches, no posters you can attach to create visually stimulating texts or even a story about the virus.

Because I was home, I used other means. My mother and brother had to take the role of being my learners, my colleagues and even my editors. Some days I had to bribe my collaborators, but it was fun, and the best creativity came out in a matter of hours. I worked hard but still had to be a daughter because supper needed to be ready on time, dishes had to be washed and the house needed to show that sane people lived here.

Working from home came with its own challenges. I was not in Port Elizabeth (PE) where the network was easy to send and receive documents, and in this way, to email my learners' work for printing. It was a touch and go adventure that left me nervous and worried. In this time of uncertainty, some of my colleagues questioned me. I took the opportunity to place our current situation in context. As an educator, we need to get to know the learners and not purely focus on the curriculum, especially for the type of learner we have at our school.

Our school is a mainstream school that serves as a special school. The school is unique because we cater to those learners with behavioural problems, though we do not exclude others. With the lockdown, learners went home for the first time in two years. Because the learners were not home for such a long time, the expectations of them working in a time like this was far-fetched. Many came from traumatic backgrounds.

I was the best fit to be in their lives due to my own traumatic experiences. I could relate to these learners. Even though I was taken away from home, my mother really was not the one who hurt me, but for my safety, I remained distant from her. That was my emotional turmoil. I had hoped, by working at this school, to restore the sense of wholeness of the children. I would even be happy if all I did was to help a child read, write and be able to express themselves.

During the lockdown, I was fine but worried about how a private school teacher got paid every month and if they were as lucky as myself being a government-paid teacher.

The whole lockdown situation started a debate in my household that woke my mother up from sleeping. My brother and I stood on opposite ends of the educational divide, screaming at each other. The issues were real. I heard parents from my rural area questioning why teachers were getting paid when they could not even send work home for the children.

I was curious about teachers who had no infrastructure or equipment to allow them to use alternative methods to deliver teaching. They had no textbooks or copying machines, let alone enough papers to write on. Maybe the parents had no data to get the work, never mind the question of having access to the Internet at any time of the day. So maybe no one will do the work that I bothered to do myself. But I will do it anyway because I can at least give them the skeleton on which to build their learning and add the fat to the bones in the years to come

Schools reopened and I could finally get the rest of the resources I needed to make teaching possible. Just as I thought I could conquer the curriculum as planned, platooning was implemented. All our lessons had to be adjusted according to a trimmed curriculum. By now, it felt like I had created enough content for two years. The year felt extremely long, and there was much uncertainty about school holidays and when the academic year would end.

I am still emotional, and more questions keep coming. I have not forgotten that I am a special schoolteacher and when I see my children again in class, I need to reassure them that they are okay. I need to remember that although the formal curriculum directs us, there is a child who has more questions than answers. The learners frequently asked questions about the Covid-19 regulations implemented in our class. It would take more than answering questions; I had to model it to them.

When school restarted, I was exhausted regardless of how many learners were kept at home, I was in need of a holiday, but the work had to be done. It was important to be practical in these times. I refrained from feeding them abstract information for assessment purposes. I completed a whole Life Orientation lesson that required me to teach about diseases and hygiene. I used background schemata and more than anything else, I allowed my learners to decide on the starting point of the lesson. I listened to where my learners wanted the lessons to start. In this way, I gained their interest and their active engagement in the lessons.

Some days were better than others. I calmed their nerves. I let them know when I did not know. I would say, "We must all go find out." I tasked them with research to explore the unknown together. I was in the position of a lifelong learner once again. So, I truly am here to restore the brokenness. Through the process of restoring, I realised my broken understanding of what teaching is all about. I learnt to survive and time ran away with me.

On most days, the early morning conversations got me closer to my learners. Our distance was regulated. So, from the comfort of my own chair and the misery of their distant tables, we would reminisce about the previous day. This exercise was important because we only saw each other on alternate days of the week. A lot happens in a day of a child.

Questions like "What is Corona?" have been replaced with questions like "How will we go to the next grade?" and "Will we pass"? I remember that question from a child who had been home for five months. The only reasonable response I could give was, "It is my job to teach you and your job to learn. If we both do our part, anything is possible."

I had hoped I answered well.

Ridwan Samodien
Kannemeyer Primary (Western Cape)

I awoke from a restless night, anxiously counting the hours, then minutes, to when I had to step up to a situation I knew little about. Donning my white PPE suit, gumboots, plastic face shield mask, a pair of gloves and a prayer, I set off for school. That was my only protective armoury: Oh Lord, I need protection, but I am not sure from what!

A stringent military protocol was dispatched to the warzone by instruction from my employers. My only protection against an unseen and little-known enemy, the virus. I was scared to the point of being petrified. I was a walking comorbidity, a word I did not know just a month ago. Flattening the curve was the new goal, even though for years I could not even flatten my stomach.

As staff members arrived, I was there, greeting them with all the false energy that I could muster. I was after all the principal, the fearless leader, guiding my staff to where they had never been before. The fear and anxiety on their faces were unmistakable. There and then, it dawned on me: this job is not for sissies. It was time to lead.

My own anxieties were no longer of any consequence. I had to show up differently and dig deep into my emotional reservoir to be of service to my staff. Their well-being was inextricably linked to my well-being. We had to be there for each other if we were going to survive this onslaught of an invisible enemy and the compliance-driven, emotionally empty instructions of our employee.

Recalling the suggestion by neurologists that fear and anxiety can cause the mind to become emotionally 'stuck' and unable to think clearly and independently, I realised that I needed to draw on my Time to Think training, which is based on the premise that the quality of everything we do depends on the thinking we do first.

Once the initial Covid-19 screening of staff had been completed, we all gathered inside the hall. With physical distancing in place, I began to create a Thinking Environment, starting with a check-in round (In a round, everyone has the turn to speak, knowing that they will not be interrupted). This was followed by rounds to reflect on the Covid-19 protocols and regulations and find creative applications for the practical implementation of the safety requirements. The rote-learning model of conditioning actually helped.

After creating the space for sharing and dialogue, anxiety levels slowly began to subside. In its place, independent and creative thinking began to surface. This continued until some members became agitated, their pent-up emotions giving way to feelings of frustration which then changed into feelings of action, as they could not wait to get started on our safety programme.

After materials had been bought, lines and dots painted, masking tape stuck on floors to show safe distances with squares on the floor, the mood of the entire staff became more positive. Activity creates progress. This intervention of spending time paying attention to each other, and practising listening, had created the conditions in which we could grow.

Together we discovered how the practice of transcendence leadership could kindle a powerful energy that would permeate every facet of school life. That spirit of transcendence had inspired a staff team that had been badly shaken. As we set up structures and created a sense of safety, the healthy organisation we designed and creatively built over the years, began to reap dividends.

With our worst fears now eased, we could now be there for each other and our parent community. We reconnected with over 90% of our parents via WhatsApp. We provided hard copies of homework to enable them to support our distant learning programme in the safety of their homes. A colleague and I registered for an online course on teaching via WhatsApp, and we assisted the rest of the team to use the platform for teaching and to clear up misconceptions using voice notes or short videos.

As news of infections and deaths amongst staff at other schools surfaced, it dampened the spirit and mood at our school. I had to dig deep and find creative ways to lift staff morale. I decided to call a 'time-out' from the compliance rules and established a dialogue circle to deal with the complex nature of what we were all experiencing.

Early in this crisis, I was told that a member of my team had tested positive for Covid-19. On hearing this scary news, I went into shock. It took me several minutes to compose myself and think about how I was going to break it to staff. With their already fragile emotions in mind, I shared the news with them gently and spent time listening as they vented their fears and concerns. Paying attention as a leader is a way of saying, "You are precious, you are appreciated, and you matter."

Although my responsibility as a principal is to also be there for the children, I found that in this time of crisis that the well-being of my staff was primary. My team and I learnt to become more resilient as we learnt to draw deep on the inner strength that was available to us in moments of need.

We also had to learn resourcefulness. Early in the lockdown, I realised that a serious financial crisis was likely to hit our school. I sent out a tweet and to my delight, but not surprised, a certain professor reached out to me. I had earlier leant how he had assisted another school in raising almost half a million rand, and I was quietly optimistic that he could do some magic for us as well.

Long story short, he reached out to his network of a few close funders and this resulted in almost R300 000 being donated to Kannemeyer Primary. This amazing intervention did not only bring financial stability to our school but emotional well-being to the leadership of the school. My fear and anxiety about the possibility that we may not be able to pay our SGB staff members subsided. I was able to focus less on finances and more on the emotional and physical health of my team.

Mabasa Alen Zimunya
Carter High School (KwaZulu-Natal)

The closure of schools scuttled our plans. It would have a ripple effect on the Annual Teacher Plans, lesson plans, assessment plans and everything else. The next workplace decision drove me very close to cardiac arrest. My school decided that we should maintain contact with our learners via cyberspace.

Teacher-pupil fraternisation on social media has been a controversial topic for a long time. Many questions have been raised on whether teachers should accept their learners as friends on social media platforms such as Facebook. I had never thought I would avail my cell phone number to my learners. I had my reservations, but begrudgingly set up a WhatsApp group for my soccer boys to facilitate ease of communication. What my school was suggesting was not exactly new. Many teachers had amicable social media contact with their learners, but I was not ready for the big shift that was being suggested. It was therefore with some trepidation that I scribbled my WhatsApp number on the board. I could not believe myself.

On lockdown level 5, everything ground to a halt. Then the flurry of cyberspace activity kicked in. It was set off by one of my learners, acknowledging and appreciating my efforts at helping my learners. More disconcerting cyberspace tendencies followed. Task after task was sent to learners via WhatsApp, learners who would not lift a finger to see to any of the tasks I gave out, learners who genuinely did not have access to gadgets that could get them connected to me, parents who were convinced that their children were being "left behind", panic-stricken learners who suddenly realised that they could not spell a particular word a minute after midnight, learners who seemed to understand everything so perfectly that they did not ask any question and the majority of learners who did not access any of the material I put up. My cell phone became a hive of activity as I desperately tried to play the educator, the counsellor, the shoulder-to-cry-on and a host of other roles that kept mutating and morphing. In the midst of all this, I was playing Dad to family thousands of kilometres away with puzzles and quizzes becoming a staple of our communication.

With my school leadership encouraging and acknowledging teachers' attempts at reaching out to learners, I discovered an unsavoury development amongst the teaching staff. We seemed to have suddenly awoken to the reality that we had to keep teaching our classes during the lockdown. The avalanche of work that we were sending to our learners seemed to be born out of some unwritten laws of a competition that cunningly pitted us against each other. There appeared to be a sudden urge to outdo each other in terms of the volume of work we dished out regardless of how much was being accomplished, let alone assimilated. The learners and their parents were roped into this and were quick to bemoan those teachers who were perceived as doing little for their classes. This came at a price for the parents as, invariably, they could not effectively monitor their children nor assist with difficult tasks. Professor Google was forced into overdrive.

The curriculum kept me awake, restless. I wanted to cover every inch as meticulously as I would have done in normal circumstances. It was a complex matter. I was not delivering 'live' cyberspace classes. It was not easy to match the pedagogical side of me to the means of delivery that I had settled for. It left me frustrated and perplexed my learners. However, we trudged on trying to cover chunks of the curriculum in as little as two WhatsApp messages. Learners were starting to rethink their choice of career paths that were so neatly laid out before the pandemic.

The extended lockdown announcement threw all my planning into disarray and made some of my efforts redundant. I felt stupid. It was painful to inform my classes that some of the work we had covered was of no use to their year mark. One of my learners did not forgive me for that.

In the flurry of activities – from marking faint or blurry essays sent via WhatsApp to responding to questions from parents who wanted to know what day it was – two developments hit me so hard that I will never be the same. One of my learners had to use a classmate to ask a question on her behalf. I picked this up later and, upon enquiry, discovered that the learner was so scared of me that she could not even use the facelessness of a cyberspace message to communicate with her teacher. I am yet to find a professional to help me deal with the PTSD (Post Traumatic Stress Disorder) this caused me. In the meantime, I find myself grinning and guffawing like a drunken clown every time I teach a particular class. The mask complicates my mission as it either saves me untold embarrassment or frustrates my attempts at being 'nice'.

The second development is diametrically opposed to the first one. I now have all my learners on my contact list, but there was a time when I did not have all of them. It was with a fearful heart that I turned to a 01:39 message from a WhatsApp number I could not place. The volume of traffic on my cell phone had drastically increased. I was taking frequent sabbaticals from that wretched gadget, but the feeling that I could be delaying a response to someone in urgent need kept gnawing at my conscience. I read the message. My world changed forever. It was not a question. It was not a complaint. It was not work for me to mark. It was not a parent who did not have a calendar.

"Sir, I just wanted to know if you and your family are ok," it read. I will keep this message forever.

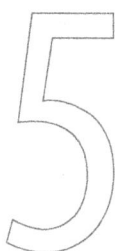

What do we learn from the teacher stories in this book?

Ten lessons for a post-pandemic school system

JONATHAN D JANSEN & THEOLA FARMER-PHILLIPS

The rich, nuanced, and inspiring accounts of pandemic teaching contained in this book have three benefits. One, they leave for the historical record a comprehensive account of how South African teachers navigated the uncertain waters of a once-in-a-lifetime pandemic. It is truly remarkable what was accomplished through the act of teaching during and after the months of lockdown. Two, they cast a harsh light on the deep inequalities that beset our school system with potentially catastrophic learning outcomes in the years ahead. We knew the inequalities were there, but this time, we could not look away. And three, they offer vital lessons for education in a post-pandemic world. That is what this closing chapter draws from the 65 beautifully composed teacher stories we were privileged to read and publish.

Lesson 1: The future is hybrid

Gone are the days of face-to-face teaching as the norm for classroom instruction. The pandemic disrupted institutional common sense – that the only way to teach is with an adult in a classroom full of children. Forced to teach children in their homes during lockdown, all kinds of inventions came to the fore, from simple WhatsApp communication to sophisticated tech platforms. In the process, teachers learnt that there are certain efficiencies that come from hybrid teaching – such as communicating about lessons (or 'admin') with learners and parents in real time. Not everything has to be done at school or carried home in heavy rucksacks.

Designed well, lessons could be done at home in ways that encourage active learning without the constraints of a crowded classroom or a 40-minute period. Smart schools, especially those who had invested in hybrid teaching before the pandemic, were the ones that sailed seamlessly between face-to-face and online learning once the lockdown happened. Sadly, there are schools that will reset to pre-pandemic pedagogies either because of a lack of resources or a shortage of initiative or the grip of habit. These are the schools that will slide further behind and be completely unprepared for future pandemics when schools close down again.

Lesson 2: The digital divide is real

Once upon a time, the world was divided between those with money, knowledge, and connections – and those without these properties. For schools, the big divide will be between the 'technological haves' and the 'technological have-nots'. Teachers in poor and working-class schools saw this and, as the stories tell, they were emotional – sometimes angry – about the persistent divide. These teachers felt helpless, for they could see the consequences of a growing, yawning gap between the education of the privileged and the poor.

The problem is soluble but not without citizen action. If unions only fight about teacher salaries, then the gap will persist. If the department limits its concerns to playing 'catch-up' for time lost, then the 'haves' move further ahead. If school leaders (principals and their teams) render themselves victims, then nothing will change. Closing the digital divide is probably the single most compelling policy and planning question to come out of this pandemic. If we lose this fight, it's over for disadvantaged schools and their precious charge.

Lesson 3: Coverage is not competence

One of the strangest things to be observed is how the curriculum pendulum swung from completely OBE (outcomes-based education) to a content-heavy CAPS curriculum. In the early days of democracy, the government pinned its hopes on a bare-bones curriculum organised around essential outcomes; teachers were trusted as professionals to give expression to those outcomes in accordance with their knowledge with adaptation to their particular contexts. Well, that idea was jettisoned in favour of an overloaded curriculum with highly prescriptive content for every teacher to follow.

Then came the pandemic, and the department realised that there was no way in which the constricted time from an extended lockdown would allow for a full-scale assessment of learning at the end of 2020. The response was the so-called 'trimmed curriculum' and a reduction in the number of accompanying assessments. We need to be careful. Some of the trimmed content was essential knowledge that needs to be taken up in the next academic year. But quite a bit of that content was redundant anyway; the curriculum spring cleaning should have happened anyway, and now it was forced upon officialdom by a pandemic.

Now is the time to bring the curriculum planners and subject experts into one room and completely revise and review CAPS to lessen the load on teachers and to make learning a lot more sensible for children. One of the most important lessons from curriculum history is that less is more; the essential skills and concepts for learning carry much more value than force-feeding children with content-heavy subject matter. Coverage is not competence.

This is also the time to introduce completely new content into the Science curriculum, such as the history of pandemics and an extended time devoted to pathogens, immunology, and vaccines. Every child must learn about technology in a much more extensive and hands-on curriculum from the earliest grades through matriculation. This is the generation that must be equipped with knowledge on the value of science and the dangers of science denialism. And to 'add' these new ideas to the curriculum means taking out much of the content that belongs in another century.

Lesson 4: Parents matter (after all)

For most schools, the lockdown caught them off-guard when it came to parent-school connections. Many teachers reported not having current or complete contact information for the parent of every child. By the way, how is this even possible? The result was then when the lockdown happened, it was not possible to instantly contact every home because the records were incomplete.

There was, however, a much bigger discovery about to be made. The partnership between parents and schools, in many cases, was non-existent. When schools called on parents to come online with or without their children, few did. Sometimes it was a matter of lack (data and devices); at the other times, it simply was disinterest. Here, too, the long shadow of our brute inequalities would become evident.

Most parents in disadvantaged communities could not help their children with learning from home. They lacked sufficient formal education; many having dropped out of school. Others were illiterate. To ask parents to be the teachers-from-home is a middle-class pipedream. There was also the reality of the social conditions of struggling communities – crowded spaces, noise, and all kinds of dysfunction. How does a child learn, even independently, in such trying conditions?

This discovery made visible by the pandemic is a call to action. The answer is not to give up on parents but to lay the groundwork for the active involvement of parents beyond the pandemic. An action agenda means investing in the education of parents in order to advance the education of children, which in turn strengthens the bond between school and home. Fortunately, there are actually existing models of parental empowerment to support learning at home. The most well-known is MathMoms, an initiative that teaches mothers-at-home Mathematics so that they can help their children learn this challenging subject. It works and more – some of the unemployed, under-educated mothers went on to become teachers themselves!

The pandemic gives us an opportunity to mend this broken relationship between parents and teachers, education at home and at school. If we take up this challenge in the department and in every school, empowering parents becomes a gamechanger, especially for children of the poor in the years beyond this pandemic.

Lesson 5: Collegial learning boosts teaching quality

Teaching is the most isolated profession, quipped someone, apart from deep-sea diving. A teacher closes the classroom door and does her or his own thing as an autonomous professional. The pandemic changed all of this. Teachers scrambled to learn the new tech platforms, often from younger, tech-savvy colleagues. Teachers called their colleagues at other schools to find out how they were teaching topics X or Y on a reduced timetable and with new technologies. Teachers went online to source content from other teachers who were demonstrating how to teach the subject. Instantly, highly successful teachers – like *Wiskunde Juffie* in this book or *Juffrou Angelique*, who reached an audience of more than 50 000 with short teaching snippets on TikTok – became celebrity teachers as others flocked to learn on their respective platforms; Likes and followers skyrocketed, much to the surprise of these expert teachers. Never before had teachers opened themselves up to collegial learning as happened during the pandemic.

With only the Grade 7s returning at one point and some teachers from that grade staying home because of comorbidities, schools asked teachers in other grades and phases to share responsibility for teaching this final grade of primary school. For some teachers this was a stretch while for others it was a unique opportunity to listen to and learn from their colleagues about how to teach a different subject in a different grade and sometimes even a different phase. There were opportunities for collegial learning at every point during and after the lockdown, and that included learning from curriculum advisors (department officials) whose status amongst many teachers turned positive as they showed up with new materials for teaching and learning.

The question is: will schools build on the momentum offered by collegial learning? That is not clear at all. Institutions like schools tend to reset after an external shock. That would be a huge disappointment since, in this case, the whole is more than the sum of the parts; that is, much more was achieved in schools than would have happened with every teacher doing their own thing, locked behind their own classroom doors. The outcome depends on leadership; that is, school leaders and district officials who understand the momentous shift in collegial learning that just happened will seek to institutionalise such interchange amongst teachers through new guidelines, incentives, and support measures within and across cooperating schools.

Lesson 6: The post-pandemic future requires different kinds of teachers

The moment lockdown first happened and the transition to some form of online learning became inevitable, there were older teachers who wondered whether they were still relevant to the profession. The demands placed on them by the new technology were experienced as onerous, leading to feelings of frustration. In general, younger teachers with pre-existing tech skills took to the new arrangements with enthusiasm. It was clear that the teaching approaches of the future would require a more agile, tech-savvy, and responsive teacher.

The shifts were subtle but significant for all teachers but especially for those prepared for their professions in another era. The foundation-phase teacher would feel the physical realignments imposed by distancing. Sitting down with groups of children on a mat was out. Moving from desk to desk to aid a slower learner was unwise. Teaching through a mask was stifling. Repeating lessons for classes split in half was tiring. The problem is that the norms themselves had changed: where once a teacher insisted that cell phones be put away (or not brought to school at all), now the teacher required the cell phone to be brought to the teaching and learning situation even if only to download course material sent home.

And then there was the new technology with all the struggles of mastery of the gadgets, connectivity and uncertainty – How do I know whether every child grasped the new concept? From behind a screen, that was impossible to gauge.

The post-pandemic teacher will have to learn a whole new range of pedagogical techniques that should result from both pre- and in-service education. Colleges and universities that prepare new teachers for the profession carry an urgent responsibility to scope the terms of a new curriculum for teacher education that is informed by what we learnt during the 2020/2021 pandemic years. No teacher can, for example, be trained without both the theory and practice of a range of new technological platforms being part of their training. The teacher already in service has to be fitted with the social and technical skills to be able to teach children in ways that build on lessons learnt from the pandemic. Practising teachers need training in *andragogy* (the concepts and methods of teaching adult learners) so that they can more effectively prepare parents for teaching children at home, now and beyond the constraints imposed by the pandemic.

The failure to completely overhaul teacher preparation and development simply means that we are postponing vital learning when the next disruption of schools happens.

Lesson 7: The district as a resource for teaching and learning

District officials are not highly regarded in many schools. They are sometimes called the post office workers of the department. The truth is, not many teachers have a high regard for their educational expertise. They are tolerated in many places and for the more activist teachers, these departmental officials still carry the stigma of the apartheid inspectorate.

The pandemic changed that image of district-level support in fundamental ways. The teacher stories in this book speak mostly of the valuable role of curriculum advisors, for example, as resource persons who brought accessible and inventive materials and tools for teachers to use during and after the lockdown. Some subject advisers went to great lengths to bring electronic materials sourced from various sites. Others jumped in and helped with school-based assessments. To be sure, there was frustration with the changing demands issued from the department, but most teachers understood this to be part of the overall uncertainty of the lockdown months.

In practice, this re-definition of the role of district-level support must be sustained beyond emergency situations. Here, too, there needs to be a reskilling of critical personnel such as your curriculum advisors so that their range of knowledge and application brings something new to the advice they give teachers. The professional advancement of the district officials is a long-delayed concern that must now be an investment priority. Once again, will the government department make this a good crisis to learn from, or will this moment of learning go to waste?

Lesson 8: Leaders matter

The stories show how school leaders emerge in a crisis. Not the one 'man' but the leadership team. When the chips are down, they show up. The pandemic split school leaders into two groups: those fully engaged in the emergency routines of mitigation and the catch-up pedagogies of the department (compliance) and those who, in addition, made time and space for caring for their people.

No story is more touching than the one of principal Ridwaan Samsodien from a Grassy Park primary school. He intuitively understands that the greater problem he faces is the spiritual, emotional, and psychological health of his staff. To keep the ship afloat, he first needs to take care of the teachers and workers who steer it. He arranges several sessions in which staff can talk and be heard and in which leaders listen. There is a readily available repertoire of team building events available to this principal from development opportunities made available by groups like Partners for Possibility, a non-profit venture that creates productive partnerships between business leaders and school leaders. The emotional infrastructure of the school is critical for successful teaching and learning.

The beauty of the stories of teacher leaders in this book is that they speak openly about their own vulnerabilities in the pandemic crisis, especially during the early weeks. They are, quite frankly, scared but know that they must project courage and give reassurance despite their own fears and doubts. That is authentic leadership – it starts with the recognition of one's own humanity, even frailty, as a source of strength. It is, of course, paradoxical but not without precedent. A well-known leader from Biblical times put it this way: "For when I am weak, then am I strong."

The teachers' stories readily refute the strong man theory of leadership – that single, heroic leader who takes the crisis by the scruff of the neck and sets the school on a steady course. That nonsense belongs in Tarzan movies. In the real life of organisations, leadership is strong in a different way in that it gains its strength from the collective. None of these schools would have survived without the combined efforts of leaders from the foundation phase coordinator to the senior matric teacher to the SMT (school management team) who had to make sense of the crisis to those looking to them for leadership.

To paraphrase Michelle Obama: a crisis does not make leaders; it reveals them.

Lesson 9: Schools do not exist for learning (only)

Some things only become clearer in a crisis – and this was a major one. What many teachers know intuitively, every teacher now knows as a bald fact. For children, school is much more than a place to learn languages or Mathematics. For many, school is a refuge from a broken home. For some, it is the one place in which a guaranteed meal will be secured. For most, it is a place for meeting and making friends, thereby adding an important dimension to learning: *how to be*. And then the harsh reality in several of our communities that the school might be the one place where children experience a loving, caring, and listening adult in their lives.

Our book *Learning under Lockdown* explains the unexpected: most children *wanted* to go back to school. They said that they missed their teachers. They longed for their friends. It was not the same 'seeing' teachers and peers online. They wanted to play, wrestle, compete, tease, share, and joke together in real school – all things that social distancing made impossible. We are only beginning to grasp the emotional consequences of the extended lockdown on children's health; those effects might be seen in the years to come.

School is a social space that teachers and children need. How often did we read in these stories the desperate need felt by teachers to hug and reassure a child as scared eyes peek above the face mask? Physical touch is so much part and parcel of the connection that teachers make with children, especially in the foundation years of primary school.

Those emotional connections in school can extend the warmth of family, but often, it substitutes for what is lacking in broken homes.

We neglect these vital functions of schools at our peril, particularly for the many children who come from precarious communities. What can and should we take from this important pandemic insight? That schools need more investments in counsellors, psychologists, and social workers who can create the conditions under which learning can flourish; in the absence of such additional personnel, the burden falls on an already overstressed teacher population.

Lesson 10: Teachers were the frontline workers

Exhaustion. It is the one word you find running through all the teacher stories, a sense of utter exhaustion. When the lockdown came, teachers sprang into action. Many said: I have never worked this hard in my life. They had to make a broken system work in many of our schools while at the same time making every effort to avoid infection. They did this even as there were 17 471 Covid cases amongst teachers and more than 1 169 teachers died as a result of the disease; and between March 2020 and February 2021, a further 1 678 teachers had died of Covid-related illness (National Income Dynamics Study, May 2021).[1] Regardless, the teaching had to be done.

All teachers worked hard and at risk to their own health. But it is important to recognise those who went beyond the call of duty. Those who physically went to find children at home or in the surrounds, who did not pitch up for an online session or had not submitted homework per the assignments sent home. Such stories in this book are heartbreaking. It threw a light on what we did not know, at least not as clearly, that there are teachers who make it their duty to bring children into learning when there are signs of them being lost to education.

What teaching from home did was to create an endless day. It is a phenomenon not yet fully understood or explained in social science research. In normal times, you leave your school or office and go home; that is the break-even if you picked up on work again later that night. Now, there was no 'break' since you were working at home. As a result, many teachers anxiously fielded questions from learners late into the night and sometimes in the early morning whenever the phone pinged.

Teachers became worried when they saw how little learning took place at home in many schools and communities. How did they notice this? The lack of development in the fine-motor skills of a Grade 1 child or the obvious gap in connecting knowledge for a History or Geography student. That is why so many stories warn about the coming crisis

---

1   NIDS-CRAM synthesis report Wave 4, page 5 [https://www.datafirst.uct.ac.za/dataportal/index.php/catalog/867].

as a result of the knowledge gap between what learners going into 2021 do not know or what they have not mastered in the truncated academic year that was 2020.

As the fog of the pandemic begins to lift, it is increasingly clear that it was the teachers who held the system together and prevented its total collapse. Those who measured their workload with hurtful comments about 'laziness' or 'sitting at home' in the lockdown either do not have children or are quite simply ignorant. What we know for sure is that the sudden lockdown of the nation and its schools could have had even more catastrophic social and educational consequences were it not for teachers and their sacrifices.

It is for this reason that we dedicate this book to those teachers who died in the struggle to advance teaching and learning in the shadow of a global pandemic.

Resources on pandemic school teaching for further reading and research

Blewett, A. (2020). Life in lockdown – teachers' stories from the COVID-19 frontline. *Teachwire*. https://bit.ly/34P93vG

Chambers, E. (2020). Lessons learnt during COVID-19 lockdown. *The Royal Society*, 14 September. https://bit.ly/3ckRUOr

Doucet, A., Netolicky, D., Timmers, K. & Tuscano, F.J. (2020). *Thinking about pedagogy in an unfolding pandemic*. An Independent report on approaches to distance learning during the COVID-19 school closures. Report written to inform the work of Education International and UNESCO, 29 March. https://bit.ly/3iiMual

Evans, C., O'Connor, C.J., Graves, T., Kemp, F., Kennedy, A., Allen, P., Bonnar, G., Reza, A. & Aya, U. (2020). Teaching under lockdown: The experiences of London English teachers. *Changing English: Studies in Culture and Education*, 27(3). https://doi.org/10.1080/1358684X.2020.1779030

Hamilton, L.S., Kaufman, J.H. & Diliberti, M.K. (2020). *Teaching and leading through a pandemic: Key findings from the American educator panels Spring 2020 COVID-19 surveys*. Creative Commons Attribution 4.0 International Public License, 2020. https://doi.org/10.7249/RRA168-2

Hoadley, U. (2020). *Schools in the time of COVID-19: impacts of the pandemic on curriculum*. RESEP Non-Economic Working Paper, Stellenbosch University, November. https://bit.ly/3fRATOc

Jaine, S., Lall, M. & Singh, A. (2020). Teachers' voices on the impact of COVID-19 on school education: Are Ed-tech companies really the panacea? *Contemporary Education Dialogue*, 18(1). https://doi.org/10.1177/0973184920976433

Majeed, Z. (2020). Teaching in a post-Covid world: Six principles for designing back to school assessments. *Oxford Policy Management*, Blog, July (Myanmar). https://bit.ly/3z68viH

Moss, G., Allen, R., Bradbury, A., Duncan, S., Harmey, S. & Levy, R. (2020). *Primary teachers' experience of the COVID-19 lockdown: Eight key messages for policymakers going forward*. Institute of Education, University College London, International Literacy Centre, June. https://bit.ly/3vWFHaG

Reimers, F., Schleicher, A., Saavedra, J. & Tuominen, S. (2020). *Supporting the continuation of teaching and learning during the COVID-19 pandemic: Annotated resources for online learning*. OECD. https://bit.ly/2RoDo11

Contributing authors

ERIN CHOTHIA-LAKAY is a graduate of the University of the Western Cape (BSc Biotechnology) with experience in the private sector as a microbiologist. Upon completion of a Postgraduate Certificate in Education, she entered the education sector and now serves as a subject head at Fairbairn College. She coordinates a cultural programme at the College in the area of dance and is an avid writer in her spare time. [orcid: 0000-0001-6986-1202]

THEOLA FARMER-PHILLIPS is a departmental head at Yellowwood Primary School in Cape Town. She serves as an advisory member of the Primary Science Programme. She is a student at the University of the Western Cape and in her free time she does content development and mentoring at the Cape Teaching and Leadership Institution. [orcid: 0000-0002-1347-7591]

JONATHAN D JANSEN is Distinguished Professor of education at Stellenbosch University. He is President of the Academy of Science of South Africa and Chairman of the Jakes Gerwel Fellowship, as well as an author and co-editor of *Schooling in South Africa: The Enigma of Inequality* (Springer, 2019). [orcid: 0000-0002-8614-5678]

DAVID J MILLAR is a Wits-trained teacher by profession and has served education in South Africa for 32 years. A master's graduate from the University of Cape Town, having specialised in education policy and planning, he is the former principal of Norman Henshilwood High School in Cape Town and the former District Director of Metro North in the Western Cape. He currently serves as Chief Executive of the National Professional Teachers' Organisation of South Africa (NAPTOSA) Western Cape. [orcid: 0000-0002-5119-6379]

www.ingramcontent.com/pod-product-compliance
Lightning Source LLC
Chambersburg PA
CBHW080603170426
43196CB00017B/2888